LEGAL ISSUES IN
PSYCHIATRIC CARE

LAURENCE R. TANCREDI, M.D., J.D.
*Fellow in Psychiatry,
Department of Psychiatry,
Yale University School of Medicine,
New Haven, Connecticut;
Former Senior Professional Associate,
Institute of Medicine,
National Academy of Sciences,
Washington, D.C.*

JULIAN LIEB, M.B., B.CH.
*Assistant Professor of Psychiatry,
Department of Psychiatry,
Yale University School of Medicine;
Director, Dana Psychiatric Clinic,
Yale-New Haven Hospital,
New Haven, Connecticut*

ANDREW E. SLABY, M.D., M.P.H.
*Assistant Professor of Psychiatry,
Department of Psychiatry,
Yale University School of Medicine;
Director, Emergency Psychiatric Service,
Yale-New Haven Hospital;
Attending Psychiatrist, Community Support Service,
Connecticut Mental Health Center,
New Haven, Connecticut*

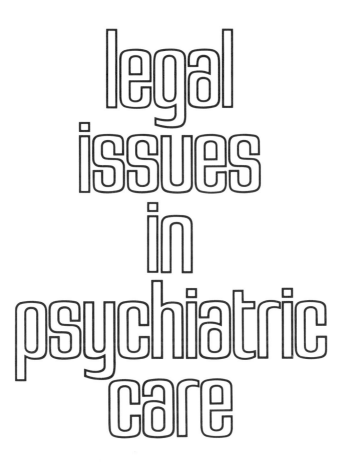

legal issues in psychiatric care

Medical Department
HARPER & ROW, PUBLISHERS
Hagerstown, Maryland
New York, Evanston, San Francisco, London

LIBRARY OF CONGRESS CATALOGING IN PUBLICATION DATA

Tancredi, Laurence R
    Legal issues in psychiatric care.

    Includes index.
    1. Mental health laws—United States. 2. Psychiatric personnel—Legal
status, laws, etc.—United States. 3. Forensic psychiatry. I. Lieb, Julian, joint
author. II. Slaby, Andrew Edmund, joint author. III. Title. [DNLM: 1.
Forensic psychiatry. W740T162L]
KF3828.T36   344'.73'044   75–8949
ISBN 0–06–142524–9

CONTENTS

PART IV THE MENTAL HEALTH PROFESSIONAL AS DEFENDANT

PART V CONFLICTS IN RESPONSIBILITY ROLES OF THE MENTAL HEALTH PROFESSIONAL

PREFACE

In the spring of 1971, a small study[1] was undertaken of mental health profession-als at a mental health center attached to a prestigious department of psychiatry to obtain an indication of how aware psychiatric clinicians were of the legal rights of patients at the time of their admission and during subsequent hospitalization. The major questions were quite direct and simply stated, as indicated below (correct answers are given in parentheses*):

1. Does the patient have a right under the Emergency Admission Statute to demand mental examination by a physician of his own choice? (Yes)

2. What consequences follow if the physician of the patient's own choosing determines that the patient is not mentally ill? (Patient must be released)

3. Are admitting physicians required to tell the patient of his legal right to mental examination by a physician of his own choice? (No)

4. Can a patient initiate termination of involuntary emergency hospitalization? (No, except for extraordinary reasons of *habeus corpus*)

5. Does the patient have a legal right to challenge the physician's decision to hospitalize him for up to 60 days? (No)

6. How long may a patient be detained after his written notice of desire to leave the hospital? (Ten days)

7. Is the patient legally entitled to be informed of release procedure? (No)

The results of this study clearly demonstrate that the mental health profession-als, who included four psychiatrists, eight psychiatric residents, and eleven nurses and psychiatric social workers, were generally unaware of a patient's legal rights at the time of admission and during hospitalization. The following tabulation lists the number of correct answers to the above listed questions:

[1]Tancredi L, Clark D (1972): Psychiatry and the legal rights of patients. Amer J Psychiat 129: 328–330
*As we will discuss in the text, the answers to these questions vary from state to state depending on local statutes. Furthermore, the laws of the state used in this study may have changed since 1971.

CATEGORY OF QUESTION	ATTENDING STAFF ($n=4$)	RESIDENTS ($n=8$)	NURSES AND SOCIAL WORKERS ($n=11$)	TOTAL ($n=23$)
Involuntary admissions				
at the time of admission				
Question 1	3	6	5	14
Question 2	2	6	6	14
Question 3	2	4	1	7
during hospitalization				
Question 4	0	0	0	0
Question 5	0	1	1	2
Voluntary admissions				
during hospitalization				
Question 6	2	5	1	8
Question 7	2	0	1	3

A psychiatric staff's awareness of the individual rights of a patient can mean the difference between incarceration or freedom. Yet, an awareness of these rights is not alone sufficient to provide a level of treatment that maximizes psychiatric care of the patient and concern for individual rights and freedom of expression. This delicate balance of responsibility is unique to issues surrounding psychiatric care.

In actual psychiatric practice, issues are rarely black or white, but generally are shades of gray. For instance, uncertainty of a patient's suicidal or homicidal potential may lead to measures by a mental health professional that compromise a patient's freedom. If a previously healthy mother of three becomes profoundly depressed at menopause and feels that she will burn in hell for eternity for having lied to her parents as a child and claims to hear the devil bringing chains to get her, she is clearly psychotic. If in her delusional state she feels she wants to kill herself to beat the devil to the draw, she must be protected and cared for in a hospital until she returns to a more normal state of mood and a rational level of thinking. But she may refuse hospitalization. Despite her delusions and irrational guilt, she may maintain the cognitive facility to state that she has the right to refuse hospitalization and the *right* to determine whether she wishes to live or die. To further complicate matters, she may be or have access to a lawyer and cite the statutes which allow her to maintain her freedom. Such a person may, if not treated appropriately, die by her own hand with her "rights on."

Comparably, another patient, thinking he is being pursued by an underworld group into which many of his close relatives have been recruited, may tell his therapist of a design to "eradicate" with God's blessing his spouse who is "out to get me." If this man's psychotherapist believes he has a moral duty to protect his patient's wife, the confidentiality of the therapist-patient relationship must be violated and the freedom of such a patient restricted until he becomes aware of the irrationality of his thoughts. Most mental health professionals and the public would agree that in such cases the patient should be protected by involuntary admission to a psychiatric hospital. The patient, however, seeing himself as a quasiordained agent of God may disagree.

The foregoing are but a few of the complex and often muddled issues confronting a mental health professional in his daily routine as healer as well as proponent of maximal freedom for personal growth. Other situations he might find himself in which are at the interface of law and psychiatry include practical considerations of certification and commitment procedures, confidentiality, a patient's rights while in the hospital, and a patient's capacity to enter into contracts or execute wills (testamentary capacity). What are the questions that must be answered in such situations? What is the "insanity defense" and how is it used? Does mental illness free a patient from blame in a case of homicide? Or does there need to be an "irresistible urge" or an "inability to tell right from wrong"? Do psychotic patients by definition not know what they are doing? What are the differences between the test developed in the Durham decision and the Model Penal Code's rule on the insanity defense? What relevance do these rules have for the practicing psychiatrist?

Legal problems may also arise in the treatment of victims of or parents responsible for child abuse. Alcoholism and other drug addictions raise problems of treatment and often involve interaction with law enforcement agencies. In a divorce proceeding a child may be asked to testify in court as to an incestuous relationship with a parent, which could easily compromise the child's emotional well-being. The indistinct area of sexual deviancy and a psychiatric clinician's inability to absolutely state that any given individual is not entirely immune to future deviancy provides another thorny area. One of the authors was recently asked by a lawyer to state that a man applying to adopt a child had "no inclination toward deviancy." Is this ever possible to assert?

Finally, a mental health professional needs to be aware not only of those areas where he may be called as witness (e.g., insanity defense, sexual deviancy, child abuse), but also of situations for which he may be called to defend himself. What is held by the various states to be inadequate care or inappropriate care? And when is an institution liable for its care standards?

There is a growing concern in the legal community to assure both that patients' rights regarding admission to psychiatric hospitals are maintained and that the level of care being provided by mental health facilities and psychiatric clinicians is of a high quality. There should obviously never need to be any significant conflict between lawyers interested in the rights of patients and clinicians interested in their treatment. The goal of both is the welfare of the individual in the area of responsible professional service. But just as lawyers concerned with the civil liberties of psychiatric patients have the moral obligation to obtain more than peripheral understanding of the nature of mental illness and its treatment, so too, mental health professionals must be aware of their obligation to know the limits of a patient's rights, the extent of the responsibility of the mental health professional, and the responsibility of the patient himself, the family, and law enforcement agencies for an individual's behavior.

In order to provide answers and guidelines for the mental health professionals dealing with the questions and situations described in the preceding paragraphs, we embarked on this volume. While we have in no way compromised on either the scope of discussion or the quality of psychiatric or legal data included, we have written the book in such a way that previous knowledge of the legal system is not needed.

LEGAL ISSUES IN PSYCHIATRY was written for use as a textbook for students in all areas of mental health—psychiatrists, nurses, psychiatric aides and social workers, and psychologists, as well as general practitioners and family specialists.

Law students and lawyers with a special interest in these issues should find the information and discussions presented here to be of particular value. When psychiatric medicolegal issues arise in medical offices or mental health clinics, a clinician may reach for this book and find ready guidelines without a morass of legal jargon. The illustrative case examples serve as springboards for discussion and provide examples which a clinician may identify as comparable to cases he has already or may in the future encounter.

In the last section we reach beyond the pragmatic concerns of clinical psychiatric practice and grapple with the questions of who should be ultimately responsible for an individual's behavior when it is either at odds with his own well-being as defined by societal norms or at odds with societal conceptions of good as they are held in the patient's subculture. The final chapter "Realignment of Roles" proposes some possible ways in which these difficult problems may obtain resolution.

L.R.T.
J.L.
A.E.S.

LEGAL ISSUES IN
PSYCHIATRIC CARE

PART **1**

MENTAL ILLNESS
AND THE LAW

A BRIEF HISTORY
1 OF PSYCHIATRY
AND THE LAW

The history of psychiatry and the law has been in effect the history of two major themes that involve the societal control of inappropriate and injurious behavior: the determination of responsibility for criminal behavior and the requirement of commitment of those who are injurious to themselves or to others in society. Both of these themes involve the reconciling of societal needs for order and stability with the individual's rights for protection against arbitrary and unconstitutional restrictions against freedom of behavior. The tension between societal needs and individual rights is ever present; the history of psychiatry and law attests to many efforts at arriving at compromises between these two strong positions.

INSANITY AND THE ISSUE OF
RESPONSIBILITY FOR CRIMINAL BEHAVIOR

The requirement of society for peace and stability has resulted in the development of the criminal law which is specifically directed at assuring that order is maintained. By convicting and sentencing those guilty of injurious conduct against others in society as well as against society at large, the criminal law attempts to deter such conduct from happening in the future, to exact retribution for the harm done to others and to rehabilitate the offenders so that they might be returned to useful and productive roles in their communities. In order to achieve these ends, the offender must be seen as morally blameworthy for his conduct. If for a variety of reasons he lacks the capacity for free choice, then the purposes of deterrence and retribution would not be served by holding such an offender responsible.

Historical Implications

Graeco Roman The notion that an individual must have the capacity for free choice in order to be held morally and legally responsible for his actions was accepted in early Greek and Roman law (Jones, 1956). The Greeks distinguished between intentional and unintentional crimes; Aristotle explicitly stated that moral blameworthiness requires that the individual be capable of free choice. He went on to assert that such capacity was lacking in the insane as well as in animals and children (Aristotle). Roman law also held that the insane offender lacked free will and was therefore incapable of voluntary action which was essential for ascribing responsibility. He was acquitted by reason of insanity but likewise was regarded as being unable to assume civil rights. He and his property were usually under the control of a guardian during the duration of his insanity. Roman law emphasized that responsibility for criminal action required the presence of a "guilty mind" in addition to an evil act (Deutsch, 1962).

Middle Ages During the Middle Ages, the insane were judged technically guilty of crimes, though often considered deserving of pardons. Much of the interest in insanity was focused on the individual's land and estate since they could be annexed by the king according to law. In certain regions of Europe, insanity was not permitted as a defense against criminal acts and was even perceived as evidence of sin and therefore punishable.

Common Law English common law gradually adopted the concept that criminal intent must be shown for an act to constitute a crime. This requirement introduced a panoply of defenses for the purpose of delineating circumstances in which intent would be absent. One of the important defenses that emerged in the early fourteenth century was impairment of mental capacity, which included insanity as well as mental retardation (Sayre, 1932). This defense did not result in acquittal by reason of insanity but rather a verdict of guilty along with a special petition of insanity which usually induced the king to grant a pardon (Wigmore, 1894). As the frequency of these pardons increased, insanity became a valid defense and was well established in the law during the sixteenth century (Hales vs Petit, 1562). By the early part of the seventeenth century, jurists and legal scholars were devising rules for determining the degree and nature of insanity that would be necessary for excusing an individual from criminal responsibility. Initially, it was held that an individual must be totally deprived of reason if he was to successfully use insanity as a defense against criminal responsibility.

Tests of Insanity

In the latter part of the seventeenth century, Sir Matthew Hale, in an effort to categorize the defenses to criminal responsibility and thereby clarify the concept of insanity, distinguished between "total" and "partial" insanity (Hale, 1736). Partial insanity, unlike total insanity, was considered to be limited to "particular discourses, subjects or applications; or else partial in respect to degree" (Hale, 1736). He concluded that because many suffering from partial insanity are not totally devoid of reason, they should be held accountable for capital crimes. He went on to propose a test for total insanity which would exempt an individual from criminal responsibility. This test stated that a person would not be held responsible if at the time of the offense he possessed mental capacity which was less than that of a child of 14 years of age. This test never gained significant usage in the courts in England, probably because it would have resulted in exonerating a large number of criminals on the grounds of insanity.

Wild Beast Test Other tests were introduced around the same time, such as the "good–evil" test which exculpated those who were unable to distinguish between good and evil—children, the insane and retarded—,but it appears that the traditional "wild beast test" predominated, certainly until the early part of the nineteenth century. This test, which is believed to have had its origins in the thirteenth or fourteenth century (Platt and Diamond, 1965), was articulated most clearly by Judge Tracy in a case occurring in England in 1724 (Rex vs Arnold). According to the terms of the test, the judge would instruct the jury much as Judge Tracy did: "If a man deprived of his reason and consequently of his intention, cannot be guilty . . . it must be a man that is totally deprived of his understanding and memory and does not know what he is doing, no more than an infant, than a brute, or a *wild beast;* such a one is never the object of punishment" (Rex vs Arnold, 1724).

"Partial" Insanity Test In 1800 a homicide occurred which ushered in a new concept of criminal responsibility, one which was based on partial rather than total insanity (the prevailing rule up until that time). James Hadfield, acting in the conviction that he had been ordained by God to undergo self-sacrifice for the salvation of the world, fired a shot at King George III in a London theater. The lawyer for Mr. Hadfield argued that the traditional language requiring total lack of memory and understanding was not sufficient to include those situations where an individual is not ravingly mad but is still unable to assume responsibility for his actions. The court accepted this expanded definition of insanity and in fact adopted the notion that delusion in the absence of frenzy or raving madness "is the true character of insanity" (Rex vs Hadfield, 1800). Hadfield was exempted from criminal responsibility because it was demonstrated that he had a delusion and that the crime in question was a direct result of that mental condition. This case not only raised to a level of acceptability the position that partial insanity is a valid defense against criminal responsibility, but more important, it advanced the notion that a single symptom of mental disorder, in this case a delusion, ought to be an appropriate defense under insanity. By shattering the prevailing theory that insanity required total raving madness, this case prefigured what was later to become a popular concept: a person may be insane in one aspect of his thinking and perfectly sound in all others.

Although acceptance of partial insanity as a defense for criminal responsibility was not widespread, the case did result in an act of Parliament which stated that when a jury concluded that a defendent should be acquitted on the grounds of insanity, the verdict should be explicitly "not guilty by reason of insanity." Furthermore, the act went on to say that in the event of such an acquittal, the accused should be kept in custody in a place and manner according to the desires of the king (Becker, 1973). For the most part, judges continued to charge the jury with finding whether the accused had knowledge of good and evil (Rex v. Billingham, 1812).

The M'Naghten Rule The M'Naghten case in 1843 resulted in a substantial change in the legal rules regarding the determination of insanity. Daniel M'Naghten attempted to assassinate the prime minister of England, Sir Robert Peel, but instead fired at and wounded his private secretary, Edward Drummond. Two days after the injury, Drummond died and M'Naghten was indicted for murder. At the trial, it was established that the accused was an extreme paranoiac beset by a complex system of delusions, one of which included the view that Sir Robert Peel was actively persecuting him (M'Naghten Case, 1843). The defendant was examined by physicians who testified at trial that he was suffering from intense delusions of persecution which had essentially left him with no peace of mind. The doctors further asserted that the delusions were not pretended but were real in terms of the perception of the defendant.

On hearing all the evidence, the chief justice charged the jury that it was their duty to determine whether the defendant "had . . . the use of his understanding, so as to know that he was doing a wrong or wicked act" at the time of the crime. The chief justice also instructed that if the jurors found that he was not "sensible" or in a sound state of mind, he was "entitled to a verdict in his favor." On the basis of this instruction and the evidence presented at trial, the jury determined that M'Naghten was to be acquitted on the grounds of being not guilty by reason of insanity.

When the verdict was received, Queen Victoria and the public were distressed over the ambiguities of the charge that was given by the chief justice. As a result the House of Lords was asked to debate the issues with the judges to define what constituted a sound mind and therefore under what conditions the insanity defense should be applied in future cases. After much debate, the House of Lords formulated what became known as the M'Naghten rule which stated that "to establish a defense on the ground of insanity, it must be clearly proved that at the time of the committing of the act, the party accused was laboring under such a defective reason from disease of the mind as not to know the nature and quality of the act he was doing; or, if he did know it, that he did not know he was doing what was wrong" (M'Naghten Case, 1843).

The importance of the M'Naghten case beyond the fact that it provided the first major test for determining insanity, was that the testimony of physicians who are experts in the field of mental disease was given special status for determining criminal responsibility. For the first time they were allowed to venture a medical opinion on events that would be reconstructed in a hypothetical form to resemble the defendant's role in the criminal act. Even though the final determination of insanity was left to the jury, physicians could now present information on whether the accused was suffering from a mentally disabling disease at the time he committed the act and if that act was causally related to the disease process.

The M'Naghten rule soon became the basic test for determining insanity both in English courts and in American courts, until recently (Annotation, 1956; Goldstein, 1970). It was particularly useful because it allowed psychiatric testimony to establish the relationship between criminal intent and the mental state of the offender in any particular case. There was much latitude for designating a variety of mental conditions as diseases, but at the same time according to the rule, the determination of mental illness in itself was insufficient to allow for an acquittal. There were, however, problems with the rule. By focusing on the offender's ability to distinguish between right and wrong, the test did not take into account the fact that an individual might know the difference between right and wrong and still be unable to control his emotional responses. By requiring proof of impairment of cognitive function, the rule precludes for consideration under an insanity plea many who suffer from serious emotional disorders.

As a result of its language, the M'Naghten rule came to be narrowly interpreted by the majority of courts. To begin with, it was viewed as requiring a lack of cognitive understanding of the difference between right and wrong. Even more importantly, the phrase "disease of the mind" was perceived by many psychiatrists to refer only to psychoses, further eliminating other emotional disturbances from consideration under the insanity plea. As a result, disenchantment grew with the ineffectiveness of the M'Naghten rule, and states began to adopt a second test for the determination of insanity; that is, the "irresistible impulse" rule (New Hampshire vs Pike, 1869). This rule emerged in response to statements made by psychiatrists who claimed that criminal acts could be committed as a result of an impulse within the person that overcomes his own intellectual awareness of the wrongness of the act.

Irresistible Impulse Test In those states where the irresistible impulse test is used as a supplement to the M'Naghten rule, the judge informs the jury that an acquittal by reason of insanity should occur if the defendant had a mental condition that prevented him from controlling his conduct even though it might be established that he knew what he was doing and that it was an unacceptable act. The addition of this rule to the M'Naghten test suggests a recognition by the law that insanity is not just impairment of knowledge alone. Mental illness or defect can so influence the individual's self-control as to impair his power over freedom of will in choosing between right and wrong behavior even though he intellectually understands the difference (Roche, 1958).

M'Naghten–Irresistible Impulse Test By the late 1950s, over a third of the states in the United States adopted the irresistible impulse test as a supplement to the M'Naghten rule (Goldstein, 1970). Criticism of this combination, however, was similar to that levied against the M'Naghten rule alone, *i.e.*, it defined too narrowly those who should be considered insane for acquittal purposes. The major objection to the combination of these tests is that there is an inadequate emphasis on the impact that unconscious motivation operating over a relatively long period of time may have on human behavior. By restricting the definition of insanity to intellectual impairment in determining right and wrong and to immediate emotional reactions, many who suffer from long-term unconscious conflicts would be excluded from special treatment under the insanity defense (Durham vs United States, 1954).

Some legal scholars, however, take issue with this objection and claim instead that the M'Naghten rule along with the control test is sufficiently flexible to encompass a very wide range of mental diseases and defects which can affect an individual's ability to control his behavior (Goldstein, 1963). Furthermore, they argue that the narrowness of interpretation of irresistible impulse is due to a literal definition of impulse that relies on an immediate response when this need not necessarily be the interpretation. Many courts have seen this test in a broader light as referring to emotional control of behavior in general.

Durham Decision Notwithstanding the validity of the objections to the combination M'Naghten and irresistible impulse tests, a major step towards an expanded interpretation of what constitutes insanity came with the decision in the Durham case in 1954 (Durham vs United States, 1954). In this decision the U.S. Court of Appeals for the District of Columbia took the position that the M'Naghten and irresistible impulse tests were indeed too narrow because they excluded from consideration those who suffer from long-term mental disorders that can influence their control over their actions. The ruling of the Durham decision excuses an unlawful act of homicide if it can be shown to be a "product" of a "mental disease or defect." The court conceived of the mind as an integrated functional unit of intellectual and emotional components and, therefore, established that an individual suffering from a mental disease could not be expected to respond to societal sanctions as a normal individual. Because of this inability to adhere to societal sanctions, such an individual should be placed in a treatment program rather than become the object of blame and punishment. As a result, to achieve a conviction under the Durham rule, the court and jury are held to the criteria of determining that the offender was not mentally ill and that his criminal act was not the "product" of his mental condition.

In the Carter case, which occurred in 1957, the U.S. Court of Appeals for the District of Columbia defined "product" to mean that the accused "would not have committed the act" except that he was suffering from the mental disease (Carter vs United States, 1957). Nevertheless, this definition grants the psychiatrist a considerably expanded role in the court for determining responsibility. He is not only called upon to establish that a mental disease or defect exists in the offender, but he must also venture an opinion as to whether or not the act was the product of the mental condition. The Durham rule considerably broadened the classes of mental illness that could be related to irresponsible behavior but failed to provide the jury with clear criteria for establishing insanity.

The major criticism of the Durham decision is that it allows the introduction at the trial of much subjective information about the accused's mental state but does not provide to the judge and jury any meaningful standards for the evaluation of the evidence about the accused's behavior in order to determine if he were impaired of emotional control and reason and should be considered insane. The concepts of mental disease or a mental defect were not defined in the Durham decision; therefore, the test of "product of a mental disease or a mental defect" includes a variety of behaviors ranging from alcoholism and narcotic addiction to the nebulous categories of the psychopathic and generally emotionally unstable personalities. The Durham decision essentially fixed no definitional limits upon the mental conditions that should qualify for special consideration under the insanity plea.

Besides being the test for insanity in the District of Columbia, the Durham decision was also adopted in two other jurisdictions—Maine and the Virgin Islands (Goldstein, 1970). However, shortly after the decision dissatisfaction with its lack of guidelines for the jury set in. Eight years after the Durham decision, the U.S. Courts of Appeals for the District of Columbia recognized that it was critical that juries be informed of the characteristics of a "mental disease or defect" so that they could understand the range of effects that such conditions would have on an individual's ability to comply with societal and legal rules. In a case occurring at that time, the U.S. Courts of Appeals explicitly defined "a mental disease or defect" to include "any abnormal condition of the mind which substantially affects mental or emotional processes and substantially affects behavior controls" (McDonald vs United States, 1962). This decision was to some extent a return to the M'Naghten rule in that it demonstrated the courts' awareness that juries need some instruction in addition to the psychiatric testimony in order to determine if an offender should be considered legally insane. Clearly the jury needed some criteria by which to judge not only the medical description of the offender's condition but also the particular effects of that process as they would be relevant to compliance with the criminal law.

American Law Institute's Test A major move away from overwhelming reliance on medical testimony fostered by the Durham test was the decision in a very recent case in the District of Columbia (United States vs Brawner, 1972). The U.S. Courts of Appeals overruled the Durham decision and adopted the rule of the American Law Institute (ALI, 1955) which had already been adopted by the other federal circuit courts of appeals. In fact, as early as 1961, the U.S. Courts of Appeals for the Third Circuit recognized the inadequacies of the Durham decision and in the Currens case adopted a test largely based on the American Law Institute's Model Penal Code to determine criminal responsibility and legal insanity (United States vs Currens, 1961). This rule, which was subsequently adopted by the District of Columbia, states that "a person is not responsible for criminal conduct if at the time of such conduct as a result of mental disease or defect he lacks substantial capacity to appreciate the wrongfulness of his conduct or to conform his conduct to the requirements of the law" (ALI, 1955). The rule further defines "mental disease or defect" to exclude "an abnormality manifested only by repeated criminal or otherwise antisocial conduct." By including this qualification, the American Law Institute sought to exclude from consideration under the insanity defense those suffering from psychopathic behavior characterized only by the fact that the person engaged in many repeated criminal activities. This last qualification of the American Law Institute's test was not adopted by the District of Columbia courts. Instead, in the Brawner case, the U.S. Court of Appeals for the District of Columbia reaffirmed the definition of mental disease or defect that was adopted in the earlier McDonald case.

The American Law Institute's Model Penal Code's version of the insanity plea is comparable to a combined M'Naghten and irresistible impulse test. It seems merely to substitute the term "appreciate" for "know" in the M'Naghten Rule and thereby encompass the functions of emotional as well as intellectual capacities for "controlling" or "conforming" conduct to legal requirements. All the federal circuit courts have adopted this test with some minor modifications, and it is gaining more acceptance by the state courts. Even though the Model Penal Code's test more closely connects the mental condition of the offender with the criminal act, there still remains some vagueness concerning the limits to what might be considered a mental disease or defect. Nevertheless, the test does seem to be a better definition of mental illness than the Durham test which essentially left the decision of what should be considered a mental disease or defect totally up to the opinions of medical experts.

In addition to these various tests for the insanity plea, there are mechanisms in the criminal law which allow the individual offender with mental illness to avoid the insanity defense and yet still be released from his conduct. There are advantages to using a legal mechanism other than the insanity defense for those who are mentally ill. Those exculpated from criminal action on the basis of insanity may be confined in mental institutions under a treatment rationale for as long, if not longer, than they would have been confined had they been judged guilty and placed in the prison system. If at trial an act can be shown to be truly involuntary —occurring during a convulsion, sleep or hypnosis, for example—then the act would not be considered criminal and the offender would be free from relying on an insanity plea. In addition to involuntary acts, self-defense and proof of coercion are valid defenses whereby the mentally ill offender can be relieved of responsibility.

Wells-Gorshen Doctrine

Two Stage Trial In California, the two-stage trial has fostered a concept called the Wells-Gorshen doctrine which allows mental illness to be introduced as a defense against criminal intent, a necessary component of many serious crimes; essentially the offender is held not guilty without relying on the insanity plea. The two-stage trial, a relatively recent development in California, is characterized first by a trial to determine whether the offender is guilty of the crime. If so, there is a second trial to establish the appropriate sentence. According to this system, proof of insanity is important in the second trial where it might, if established, result in having the offender placed in a mental institution rather than a prison. The Wells–Gorshen doctrine, however, allows information on the mental condition of the offender to enter into the first stage of the trial, at which time the court and jury are deciding whether the offender is even guilty of a crime. This doctrine is sufficiently broad to allow the introduction of evidence of a mental condition whenever an offender is charged with a crime that requires the presence of a guilty mind, such as murder or armed robbery. It can result in a reduced sentence.

The history of the development of tests for the determination of insanity shows that the concept of criminal responsibility is complicated. Various tests, such as the M'Naghten rule, the irresistible impulse test, and most recently the Durham decision and American Law Institute's test, have been proposed; each has its own emphasis on what is important about the mental condition of the offender and what role psychiatric testimony should play. A great number of courts, however, are more frequently taking the position that the exact wording of the charge to the jury or the name of the test is essentially unimportant. In the final analysis, any rule can be interpreted either broadly or narrowly, and the critical issue is whether the charge contains the following three essential considerations—an assessment of the offender's intellectual capacities to determine right from wrong and to comply with societal and legal sanctions, an assessment of his volition from the standpoint of whether he desired to commit the crime, and a consideration of his emotional capacity to control his own behavior (Goldstein & Katz, 1963).

Psychiatry in Criminal Responsibility

Brigg's Law One other landmark event is important in the development of the role of psychiatry in determining criminal responsibility: the passage of the so-called Briggs law of Massachusetts in 1921. This law states that a person indicted for a capital offense or for any offense more than once shall be examined "with a view to determine his mental condition and the existence of any mental disease or defect which would affect his criminal responsibility . . ." (Briggs). This was the first statute enacted in the United States that established an essentially automatic pretrial mental examination of certain classes of criminal offenders. By using state-appointed psychiatrists, examinations are expected to be impartial and the trials free of the confusing testimonies of psychiatrists representing the defendant and those representing the prosecution. Because the Briggs law requires an automatic examination of certain classes of offenders, often underlying mental or psychiatric features which may have otherwise gone unnoticed are discovered. Many other states now have legislative provisions which authorize pretrial psychiatric examinations of similar classes of offenders. Most of these statutes allow the trial judge to use his discretion in determining whether such an examination should be made.

The Briggs law and similar provisions for pretrial psychiatric examinations have not precluded the testimony of expert psychiatrists called by the defendant or the prosecutor at the actual trial. The questions to be answered in a pretrial psychiatric examination involve determining the offender's mental condition, his competency to stand trial, whether he is criminally responsible for his acts and finally if he qualifies for civil commitment. The Briggs law and similar statutes have resulted in a unique role for the psychiatrist—the examination of felons and the recommendation of appropriate treatment.

CONFINEMENT FOR PSYCHIATRIC TREATMENT

Until the latter part of the eighteenth century, there were no statutory provisions for the commitment of the mentally ill. This did not mean, however, that the mentally ill could not be deprived of their liberty. In fact, common law during the early colonial period followed English decisions; those considered dangerous to others were arrested. There were no hospitals in this country until the latter part of the colonial period, and the mentally ill, paupers, and criminals were disposed of in jails and in poorhouses.

Around the 1780s, various states enacted legislation which explicitly provided for the lawful confinement of those who suffered from "lunacy" or were otherwise so "furiously mad" as to be harmful to others. Such legislation usually required that two or more justices of the peace make the decision for apprehending a mentally ill person for the purpose of safely locking the patient in a secure place (Laws of New York, 1788). Despite the fact that hospitals and other asylums for the mentally ill constructed during the latter part of the eighteenth and early part of the nineteenth century considerably expedited the commitment of the insane, no specific laws concerning commitment procedures, particularly legislative safeguards protecting the personal liberty and civil rights of these patients, were enacted until the middle of the nineteenth century. [Before such laws were enacted, the insane were often committed to a variety of institutions—including poorhouses and prisons, as well as hospitals—by friends, relatives or public officials without regard to their civil rights.]

During the early part of the nineteenth century commitment was accomplished mainly on an informal basis. There were, however, some attempts to limit the extent to which the mentally ill were placed in prisons rather than in hospitals; some states actually forbade confining the insane in penal institutions. Others restricted such confinement to short periods of time. For example, in New York, an act passed in 1827 stipulated that the indigent insane must be sent to the Bloomingdale Asylum in New York City or to houses for the poor (Deutsch, 1962)

Civil Rights

Oakes Case In 1845 the case of Josiah Oakes was of particular significance because it attracted national attention to the problems of the civil rights of the insane. Oakes petitioned the court to release him from confinement, claiming that his family had committed him to an asylum without justification. The chief justice of the Massachusetts Supreme Court denied this request and affirmed that the confinement of a mentally ill patient should continue as long as it is required for the patient's own safety or for that of others and that this is the "proper limitation." According to some, this decision by Chief Justice Shaw was among the most important decisions involving the insane in this country, because it established the foundations for justifying and limiting the extent of confinement of mental patients. It is further posed that this decision was "probably the first time that the therapeutic justification" for confinement was decided in a court in this country (Deutsch). Though it could be argued that the Josiah Oakes case was not proposing therapeutic justification for restraining the mentally ill (Kittrie, 1971), nonetheless, a discernible trend started around that time toward the broadening of reasons for commitment of the mentally ill. This expansion has now reached the point where in many states the commitment laws explicitly justify commitment on the basis of "need for treatment" which includes not only treatment for mental illness but also for alcoholism and drug abuse.

Packard Case The case of Mrs. Packard, which took place in the mid nineteenth century, was another major milestone in the evolution of involuntary commitment legislation in the United States. On the petition of her husband Mrs. Packard was committed for a period of about three years to a state mental institution in Illinois. Ultimately released, she claimed that she had been victimized by her husband and was quite sane when committed to the hospital. Upon release she launched an nationwide campaign for the enactment of protective legislation to benefit the insane. Her successful campaign resulted in changes of various commitment laws to include such important safeguards, already present in criminal law, as notice to the patient that the petition has been filed for commitment, a fair hearing on the issue and finally the right to a jury trial (Kittrie, 1971). In some states these procedural safeguards have been modified so that under emergency conditions patients may be committed without a judicial hearing simply on the establishment of medical need.

The development of commitment legislation has been for the most part left up to each state. As a result, there is little uniformity across the country regarding involuntary commitment to mental institutions. Although these procedures vary widely, there appear to be mainly four bodies for effecting involuntary hospitalization: a court, an administrative tribunal, the hospital itself and two physicians. The majority of states require hearings before a judge who has the power to commit the patient. Some of these states also specifically provide for jury trial if the patient requests it or if the judge feels it to be essential. Many states allow for nonjudicial commitment through hearings by administrative tribunals or through a decision by the hospital. In at least thirty states involuntary commitment may be effected merely with an application or sworn petition by a relative, friend or state official along with medical certificates signed by one or more physician indicating that the patient should be committed (Overholser and Weihofen, 1946). Shortly after Mrs. Packard's campaign in the 1860s, commissions on lunacy were established in various states. The function of these commissions initially was to closely monitor mental institutions, and to some extent these commissions reduced the fears and concerns of the public regarding the rights of the insane and the possible coercion of sane individuals into institutions. The functions of these commissions have expanded to the point where they now have complete administrative control over the state hospital system as well as involvment in the inspection of the various mental institutions (Deutsch, 1962; Williams, 1915).

We have been examining the development of involuntary commitment, resorted to when the patient does not request psychiatric treatment through hospitalization. It is particularly interesting that there were no provisions in the United States for voluntary hospitalization to public institutions until the end of the nineteenth century (Overholser, 1924). Voluntary admissions were discouraged except when patients were severely disordered because many states were concerned about the expenditures of money that would be necessary to care for many admissions. Some of the earlier laws limited voluntary admission to patients who could pay for care (Dewey, 1913).

By the early twentieth century, however, the emphasis was on preventive psychiatry through early diagnosis and treatment; states began to alter their policies and allow voluntary admissions. All states now permit voluntary hospitalization whereby patients may apply directly to a hospital for care. In many states there are no requirements for a judicial hearing or even for a medical certification when a patient voluntarily requests admission. Once hospitalized, however, the patient often loses important legal rights to property and personal freedom just as the involuntarily committed patient does.

Recently the trend has been toward both voluntary admission and temporary commitment for observational purposes. Short-term commitments usually last for thirty days to determine the mental condition of the patient. The patient may be committed for diagnostic purposes on the basis of medical certification alone without the requirement of other legal safeguards. At the end of the period of observation, the patient is usually released unless the physician or hospital authorities initiate more formal procedures for involuntary commitment.

Despite the progress in this country toward more effective protections against indiscriminate detention and involuntary commitment of the mentally ill, England recently passed a new Mental Health Act which provides little, if any, important safeguards. According to this act, an insane person may be hospitalized for indefinite periods of time simply on the recommendation of two private physicians without the procedural safeguard of a hearing by a court or an administrative tribunal. In addition, this act authorizes compulsory hospitalization of patients afflicted with mental illness, mental subnormality, and a variety of psychopathic disorders—concepts which are not clearly defined in the act (Kittrie, 1971).

Because the most common involuntary commitment in this country has been for an indeterminate period of time, the issues pertaining to when a patient should be released have been very important. This decision has usually rested on the hospital authorities' determination that the patient has recovered, that treatment in an institutional setting is no longer necessary or beneficial, or the patient is not harmful to himself or others. Legally commitment must end when the patient is no longer insane, but this might require a legal procedure often referred to as a habeas corpus proceeding. The patient himself, a relative, a friend, or any other interested party, such as a social agency, has the right to apply for "a writ" of habeas corpus to establish the legality of continuing confinement. Partial discharge has been available in the form of furloughs which are usually trial visits of the patient to a private home to determine his ability to return on a permanent basis to the community.

There has been a trend in recent years towards the justification of commitment of the mentally ill on the basis of therapeutic reasons. Many states contain provisions similar to those in the Virginia code which permit confinement of the mentally ill where it is necessary for their "safety and benefit to receive care and treatment" (Virginia Code, 1966). This justification for commitment of the mentally ill is also used for persons with other "behavioral" disorders, particularly drug addiction, alcoholism and sexual psychopathic personalities.

The first of these, drug addiction, is seen as a symptom of an underlying personality malfunction rather than a disease in its own right. The threat of punishment through the traditional criminal system has not been shown to control drug addiction effectively or to increase significantly the ability of the drug addict to conform to the standards of society and the law.

As early as the mid-1920s, the Supreme Court of the United States accepted the theory that narcotic addiction was a disease and that addicts were actually sick individuals (Linder vs United States, 1925). This theory was reiterated in a Supreme Court decision in the early 1960s which held that not only was addiction an illness but also that it would be violating the safeguards in the Bill of Rights to penalize individuals simply for being drug addicts (Robinson vs California, 1962). As a result of this perception of drug addiction, civil commitment for treatment of addicts became an alternative to imprisonment. Over thirty states have provisions for commitment of those suffering from narcotic addiction. An addict involuntary committed to a treatment institution is usually brought before a judicial hearing, and he is often confined either to a state mental institution or a specialized program until he is considered cured or substantially improved, at which time he is released. A troublesome feature of most state statutes providing for involuntary commitment of narcotic addicts is that they do not explicitly define the extent of addiction that would call for involuntary hospitalization. There seems in recent years to be a move towards voluntary therapeutic commitment for drug addiction (California Welfare and Institution Code, 1966; New York Mental Hygiene Law, 1966).

Involuntary commitment procedures for the treatment of alcoholism also exist in nearly thirty states, most often as provisions related to involuntary commitment of the mentally ill. Under most of these laws, an alcoholic can be voluntarily admitted or involuntarily committed for an indeterminate period until he either improves sufficiently or is cured. Similar to the decisions characterizing narcotics addiction as an illness, there have been recent cases which have classified chronic alcoholism as a medical condition (Driver vs Hinnant, 1966; Easter vs District of Columbia, 1966). In these cases the courts determined that chronic alcoholism is a condition that actually destroys the individual's control over his will. As a result, he cannot be held responsible for the crime of public intoxication. and should therefore not be punished by imprisonment or fine. These decisions, however, did not exculpate the chronic alcoholic because of his lack of free will for other criminal activities, but rather these cases gave impetus to the view of alcoholism as a medical problem requiring a therapeutic solution. Consequently, justification was established for including the chronic alcoholic in a treatment and rehabilitation program through involuntary commitment. (Hutt & Merrill, 1969)

The use of the medical model as a means of controlling deviant and unacceptable behavior has also been extended to those classed as psychopaths or sexual offenders. Statutes providing for commitment rather than imprisonment of the sexual offender emerged in the 1930s and 1940s and were reviewed by the Supreme Court which upheld the provisions for civil commitment of these deviants. (Minnesota ex rel vs Probate Court, 1966).

Epileptics also are often subjected to involuntary commitment. These patients are vulnerable to commitment in mental hospitals in nearly 20 states despite the fact that medical experts argue strongly that epilepsy is not a mental illness but a controllable physical abnormality.

Finally, with regard to commitment of the mentally ill and others in our society, there has been a gradual shift from the traditional notion of confining those who are dangerous to themselves and others toward a therapeutic justification more closely tied to the concept that these conditions are illnesses (Kittrie, 1971). There was a move following the Packard campaign toward developing legal safeguards for those involuntarily committed; judicial hearings and notice to the patient and his family of an impending commitment are mandatory according to many state statutes. But presently there appears to be a shift away from such safeguards. Only a few of those states which provide for commitment through a judicial process actually require that a hearing be conducted (Kittrie, 1971). The move seems decidedly in the direction of expansion of the use of the medical model in the control of behaviors that are considered inappropriate and unacceptable to society.

Right to Treatment

Rouse Case Before completing this short history of law and psychiatry, it is important to mention the current interest in right to treatment. This concern has emerged from the growing realization that many who are institutionalized for mental illness do not actually receive adequate medical treatment to regain their health and to return to their communities. The landmark case that introduced this issue of adequate psychiatric treatment occurred in the District of Columbia in 1966 (Rouse vs Cameron). Charles Rouse was brought to trial for carrying a dangerous weapon, which in the District of Columbia is a misdemeanor with a maximum sentence of one year if the offender is convicted. Instead of being convicted and sent to jail, Rouse was found not guilty by reason of insanity. Because of this determination he was committed to St. Elizabeth's Hospital for treatment. Four years later a habeas corpus petition was filed. Judge David Bazelon, speaking for the U.S. Court of Appeals for the District of Columbia, stated that involuntary commitment is imposed because it is assumed that the criminal offender requires treatment for a mental condition. When treatment was not given, as in the case of Rouse, who was confined three years more than had he gone to jail, the court held that the individual had been deprived of his basic rights. The Rouse case also determined that treatment must adhere at least to minimum professional standards and be appropriate to the patient's needs (Halpern, 1969).

An important decision occurred in 1970 in Alabama when the Federal district court decided that individuals involuntarily confined in institutions for the mentally ill have a constitutional right to adequate treatment and living conditions.

This case resulted in the setting of minimum standards for care including staffing patterns, physical facilities, and nutritional requirements (Wyatt vs Stickney, 1972). Already the rights of those confined in mental institutions have been expanded to include compensation for the work that patients perform in state mental hospitals as well as the right to receive appropriate education, particularly important for mentally and socially handicapped children. There will, no doubt, be many more cases focusing on the rights of the mentally ill and mentally retarded who are confined in state and private institutions.

REFERENCES

ALI Model Penal Code, (1955) Section 4.01 (1) (Tent Draft No 4)

Annotation, (1956) 45 American Law Reports 2, 1447

Aristotle: The Nichomachean Ethics. Book 3, Chapter 1

Becker R (1973): The historical background. Psychiatr Ann 3:8

Birnbaum M (1969): A rationale for the right. Georgetown Law J 57:752

The Briggs Law, (1932) Mass Gen Laws c 123, Section 100A, (Ter Ed)

California Welfare and Institution Code, (1966) Section 3100 (West)New York Mental Hygiene Law, (1966) Sections 200–217 (McKinney Supp)

Carter vs United States, (1957) 252 F 2d 608 (DC Cir)

Deutsch A (1962): The Mentally Ill in America. New York, Columbia University Press

Dewey R (1913): The jury law for commitment of the insane in Illinois. Am J Insanity 69:571

Dix G (1970): Mental illness, criminal intent and the bifurcated trial. Law Soc Order 1970:559

Driver vs Hinnant, (1966) 356 F 2d 761 (4th Cir)

Durham vs United States, (1954) 214 F 2d 862 (DC Cir)

Easter vs District of Columbia, (1966) 361 F 2d 50 (DC Cir)

Fingarette H (1972): The Meaning of Criminal Insanity. Berkeley, University of California Press

Frankel M (1966): Narcotic addiction, criminal responsibility, and civil commitment. Utah Law Rev 1966:581.

Glueck S (1966): Law and Psychiatry. Baltimore, Johns Hopkins Press

Goldstein A (1970): The Insanity Defense. New Haven, Yale University Press

Goldstein J, Katz J (1963): Abolish the insanity defense—Why not? Yale Law J 72:854

Hale vs Petit, (1562) 75 Eng. Rep. 387 (KB)

Hales M (1736): Pleas of the Crown. London, Nutt & Gosling, pp. 29–49

Halpern C (1969): A practicing lawyer views the right to treatment. Georgetown Law J 57:782

Holdsworth W (1942): A History of English Law. 5th Ed., Vol. , Boston, Little Brown

Hutt P, Merrill R (1969): Criminal responsibility and the right to treatment for intoxication and alcoholism. Georgetown Law J 57:835

Jones JW (1956): The Law and Legal Theory of the Greeks. Oxford, Clarendon Press

In Re Josiah Oakes, (1845) 8 Law Rep 122 (Mass)

Kittrie N (1971): The Right to Be Different. Baltimore, Johns Hopkins University Press Note: Kittrie is quoting Deutsch and feels that the Josiah Oakes case provides no clear expression of the therapeutic justification for restraint of the mentally ill.

Linder vs United States, (1925) 268 US 5

Lindman FT, McIntyre DM (eds) (1961): The Mentally Disabled and The Law. Chicago, University of Chicago Press

McDonald vs United States, (1962) 114 US App DC 120, 312 F 2d 847 (En banc)

Mental Health Act, (1958) 7 and 8 Eliz 2, c 72

M'Naghten Case (1843): House of Lords, 1843, 8 Eng Rep 718 (HL)

Minnesota ex rel Pearson vs Probate Court, (1940) 309 US 270

Nason vs Bridgewater, (1968) 233 NE 2d 908

New Hampshire vs Pike, (1869) 49 NH 399 (Irresistible-impulse often referred to as New Hampshire Decision)

New York Laws, 1788, Chapter 31. See: "An Act for Suppressing Rogues, Vagabonds, Common Beggars and Others Idle, Disorderly and Lewd Persons," Laws of Massachusetts, 1797.

Overholser W (1935): History and operation of the Briggs Law of Massachusetts. Law and Contemporary Problems 2:426

Overholser W (1924): The voluntary admissions law: Certain legal and psychiatric aspects. Am J Psychiatry 3:475

Overholser W, Weihofen H (1946): Commitment of the mentally ill. Am J Psychiatry 102:762

People vs Wells, (1949) 33 Cal 2d 330, 202 P 2d 53 People vs Gorshen, (1959) 51 Cal 2d 716, 336 P 2d 492

Platt, AM, Diamond, BL (1965): The origins and development of the "wild beast" concept of mental illness and its relation to series of criminal responsibility. J Hist Behav Sci 1:355

Rex vs Arnold, (1724) 16 How St Tr 684

Rex vs Billingham, (1812) 39 How St Tr 722 (KB)

Rex vs Hadfield, (1800) 27 How St Tr 1281 (Kings Bench)

Robinson vs California, (1962) 370 US 660 Congress passed act to establish new treatment centers at Lexington, Kentucky, and the other at Fort Worth, Texas. This act is the Act of January 19, 1929, 45 Stat. 1085, (ch. 82) (1929).

Roche P (1958): The Criminal Mind. New York, John Wiley and Sons

Rouse vs Cameron, (1962) 373 F 2d 451

Sayre F B (1932): "Mens Rea." Harvard Law Rev 45:974

Smith vs United States, (1929) 36 F 2d 548 (DC Cir)

United States vs Brawner, (1972) 471 F 2d 969

United States vs Currens, (1961) 290 F 2d 751 (3rd Cir)

Virginia Code, (1966) Section 37–1–1(1) (Supp)

Wigmore JH (1894): Responsibility for tortious acts. Harvard Law Rev 7:315

Williams F (1915): Legislation for the Insane in Massachusetts, Boston Smithsonian Press

Wyatt vs Stickney, (1972) 344 F Supp 373, 344 F Supp 387. Case is still in progress on appeal from the Federal District Court level in Alabama.

2 THE PATIENT–FAMILY– PSYCHIATRY– LAW INTERFACE

Psychiatry and law share many features. Both are concerned with the way people relate, the obligations and responsibilities people assume and the problems that emerge from those human relationships. Both have also been vested with certain societal duties and expectations that influence the way they function in their service to people. Mental health workers and lawyers are bound by codes of ethics which, among other requirements, place primary duty on meeting the needs of patients or clients.

In caring for a patient, the mental health worker must often protect that patient's interest even under circumstances where it would be valuable to the family or the society at large if he revealed information given to him in confidence. Similarly, the lawyer often finds himself in the position of defending clients who he may reasonably suspect have committed criminal acts. These requirements are imposed on mental health and legal professionals not because society wishes to protect the blatant criminal or the promiscuous wife undergoing divorce and demanding child custody, but because in the vast majority of situations that involve psychiatry and law, adherence to codes of ethics has been shown to be highly beneficial in treating patients or protecting clients, most of whom have not participated in crimes or deception.

There are significant differences between law and psychiatry. Law has been constructed to prevent and account for injuries that are incurred through direct intentional acts or through negligent conduct. To prevent injuries, a complex network of regulations prohibiting certain activities in human interaction has been developed which controls a variety of transactions in business and public affairs, in agreements among people such as contracts for buying and selling property, for establishing wills, and for engaging in such intimate personal acts as marriage and divorce. In its function to account for injuries that have occurred, law provides a forum—the court—for determining responsibility and punishing the offender with fines or imprisonment.

Psychiatry, on the other hand, is concerned more with the way behavior manifests itself than with the outcomes of that behavior. Using the medical model based on the distinction between sickness and health, psychiatry describes certain classes of behavior as mental illness. For example, attempted suicide, prostitution, sexual deviance and drug abuse are considered unhealthy behaviors to be handled much the same way the internist deals with diabetes; that is to say, psychiatric intervention is directed at returning the patient to a near-normal state. The primary function, therefore, of the mental health worker is to treat and care for patients who manifest aberrant behavior. Unlike the law, psychiatry has not been charged with the task of enforcing rigid societal standards to which all must conform, but rather the task of caring for those who are suffering from mental illness and unable to conform. However, as we will learn shortly, psychiatry has assumed a societal control function—perhaps not as powerful as the law, but nearly as effective.

In contrast to mental health workers, lawyers can be either agents of society or of an individual client. As an agent of society, the prosecuting attorney is entrusted with preserving order in the social system by convicting those responsible for disruption of that order. The defense attorney also receives his authority from society which enables him to defend the presumably innocent defendant from the unjust accusations of society as set forth in the declaration of the prosecuting attorney. Lawyers can assume both roles because law is concerned, above all, with the determination of truth. The adversary system, which sets in opposition two lawyers defending different interests, allows for the optimum ferreting out of information about an injury so that the judge and jury can arrive at a decision of guilt or innocence.

As we have already suggested, psychiatry also plays a role in society's control of undesirable behavior. Although its major purpose is to provide patient care by viewing particular behaviors as manifestations of mental disease, psychiatry reinforces the mode of behavior of the majority of the population. For example, until recently, homosexuality had been classified as a disease and is still considered to be by many psychoanalysts in this country. By classifying homosexuality as an illness, psychiatry was influenced by the prevailing societal mores giving preference to heterosexual conduct. Hence, the patient seeking psychiatric help for homosexuality was treated with the hope of achieving the acceptable sexual behavior—heterosexuality.

But even more significant than psychiatry's role in enforcing societal standards of conduct is its useful and important social function in the handling of the psychotic patient. It possesses authority conferred by the laws of the states to initiate immediate confinement (involuntary commitment) of those who could be harmful to themselves or others.

Even though law and psychiatry are both concerned with interpersonal relationships, they do not necessarily function in harmony when concerned with similar problems. The two can interact by being complementary or antagonistic to each other.

There are two major areas where law and psychiatry are in agreement. The first of these is in the control of so-called victimless crimes—like sexual deviance involving consenting adults or marijuana usage—where there is no objective evidence of injury. Here the law is acting primarily on the basis of psychiatric opinion that such behavior is unhealthy. Because in many of these crimes no victims can be identified, the law is actually controlling the behavior itself. In effect, psychiatry has adopted societal values and norms in its definition of these diseases, thus justifying their control by the law. Besides the victimless crimes, law and psychiatry are in accord in the treatment of the psychotic patient. The law facilitates the confinement of these patients by empowering psychiatrists to commit such patients even against their wishes.

The second area where law and psychiatry work together concerns issues of responsibility, particularly where the criminal is insane. The lawyer relies heavily on the expertise of the psychiatrist to determine whether or not a criminal could be held responsible for his behavior. If on examination the psychiatrist determines that the criminal is insane, he will not be brought to trial for his offenses until he has undergone sufficient treatment for his mental condition. Even when he stands trial for his acts, the introduction of evidence concerning his capacity to be responsible for those offenses can significantly influence the court's decision as to his guilt or innocence. It is important to recognize that concepts like "insane" and "legal commitment" are predominantly legal, not psychiatric terms. The psychiatrist is not the person who decides whether an individual was insane when he committed an act or whether a psychotic person should be legally committed for a period of treatment. The role of the psychiatrist in the determination of "insanity" and prudence of "legal commitment" remains an advisory one. The psychiatrist's contribution consists of describing the mental condition of the individual and possibly giving his opinion as to whether or not this person could have been responsible for his actions. Then the prosecuting attorney usually decides on the basis of this information whether or not the presumed criminal should stand trial, and in the event of a trial, the judge and jury determine whether a criminal should be considered not guilty on the basis of "insanity." The psychiatrist does not decide on insanity or legal commitment for these are legal concepts which are left for final determination to lawyers, judges and juries. Nonetheless, in making such decisions, the psychiatrist and lawyer work together, one in an advisory role and the other making the final decision as the representative of society.

There are other situations where lawyers and psychiatrists come into conflict. Although both groups feel that certain behaviors should be controlled, such as drug addiction and sexual deviance, they may differ on how individual offenders should be handled. Psychiatrists, in general, want to keep people who are sick out of the hands of prosecuting lawyers who will try to involve such individuals in the criminal process. For instance, many psychiatrists would prefer to treat a drug addict themselves, rather than subject him to the penalties of criminal law. A lawyer, on the other hand, is more likely to be concerned with the fact that an infraction has been committed against society and will be motivated to exact justice through the criminal process—the determination of guilt by the court or jury and subsequent penalties.

In addition to conflicts that can arise from the way lawyers and psychiatrists choose to handle individuals who engage in unacceptable conduct, the two may conflict when a patient's rights are concerned. Lawyers are particularly sensitive to the right of individual citizens to be free from detainment or incarceration without the due process of law. A psychiatrist has the power, to varying degrees depending on state laws, to detain an individual anywhere from 72 hours to 60 days in a hospital if he determines that because of mental illness, the patient is harmful to himself or to others. This power of detainment can create problems, particularly when the patient demands release and enlists the assistance of a lawyer; the lawyer is inclined to demand evidence that that patient should, in fact, be detained in the mental health facility. A court process may be required to determine if the patient should be detained for medical reasons.

In conjunction with the individual's right to be free from detainment without legal action, lawyers are also concerned with the patient's right to treatment. This issue is particularly important when a criminal enters a mental institution for treatment either before standing trial or following court determination of not guilty by reason of insanity, for there have been recent cases where such patients have brought actions against mental health facilities for not providing sufficient treatment. Besides being concerned with the inadequacies of the facilities, lawyers may also come into conflict with psychiatrists where issues of inadequate or inappropriate professional treatment are raised.

In addition to the psychiatrist and the lawyer, the family also has an important role in determining what happens to mental patients. Often the family is responsible for bringing the patient to the psychiatrist. If the psychiatrist decides that the patient should be medically committed to prevent harm to himself or to others and the patient does not voluntarily agree, the family's consent may be sufficient to allow the psychiatrist to commit him at least for a period of observation. Various motivations may underlie the family's decision to bring the patient to a mental health facility, but for the most part, families are interested in the well-being of other family members. However, one can conceive of various situations where families might use the mental health system to dispose of unwanted family members in a somewhat acceptable social manner. A promiscuous, drug-abusing, adolescent girl or a senile grandparent might be the victims of such family decisions.

Furthermore, placing a family member in a mental health institution can be a way of achieving personal gain for other members of the family. The mentally ill are often denied the right to make contracts and to either make or alter wills, in which cases it might be advantageous to the family to place a member in a situation where he effectively loses important legal rights over his property. And lastly, the mental health system might be used as a way of dealing with domestic problems. A wife or a husband might view committing a spouse to a mental institution as more expedient than divorce, or even a reason for divorce. Because of the ease with which divorces are obtained at the present time, the use of the mental health system for these purposes is probably limited to situations where a spouse might find it more desirable to avoid divorce, and at the same time get rid of an unwanted partner. Because the reasons for family decisions regarding the commitment of other family members are not always for the patient's benefit, psychiatry and law occasionally collude to help the family achieve nefarious ends.

Conflicts between psychiatrists and lawyers concerning various aspects of patient care are inevitable. By the same token, it is apparent that neither of these professionals is fully aware of the other's responsibilities and duties both to society and to patients or clients. A greater understanding of the way psychiatrists and lawyers function in the care of patients would result in minimizing some of the conflicts that occur between these two groups and at the same time allow for greater concentration on working together for the patient's rights and needs. The emphasis of both groups of professionals should be directed primarily toward the medical and legal requirements of the patient rather than the desires of the family or those of other societal institutions.

By virtue of the complicated nature of mental health and law, there are bound to be conflicts in the roles that these professionals must assume—on one level serving the needs of society for order and to some extent conformity, and on another, protecting the legal rights and health of the patients. It is particularly important that both the psychiatrist and the lawyer learn to understand how the two may work complementarily or antagonistically in their dealings with mentally ill patients. It is hoped that once these points of interaction are understood, there might be a better awareness of their sometimes conflicting roles so that the care of the patient becomes their common goal.

The following are legal issues which will be discussed in greater depth in subsequent chapters of this book.

THE RIGHTS OF THE PATIENT

At various times during the course of treatment, patients have rights that insure a certain standard of care, the confidentiality of personal information, their being informed of medical procedures, and termination of treatment if they so desire.

The Right to Psychiatric Treatment

Recently there have been several court cases which have dealt with the adequacy of treatment in mental health institutions. This issue is particularly important when it involves a person who is placed into a mental health institution by the court to be treated prior to court trial for an alleged offense. There have been instances where individuals awaiting trial have been placed in mental institutions for several years and have received little or no psychiatric treatment. Besides those awaiting trial, the courts have also been concerned with offenders who have been judged not guilty by reason of insanity and placed in mental institutions for treatment. A recent case in Alabama has extended the concern of the court even to those not subject to court order with a decision that states that all patients confined in mental institutions have a constitutional right to treatment. The court proceeded to set standards for what it considered minimum treatment in such institutions, from staffing patterns to the requirements for programs in vocational education.

Certification and Commitment Procedures

The certification of patients as mentally ill and the subsequent commitment of these patients either voluntarily or involuntarily is regulated by the laws of individual states, and these regulations vary widely. In some cases they restrict considerably the power of psychiatrists to commit involuntarily patients for long periods of time. Certification and medical commitment may be initiated by one or more physicians who do not need to be psychiatrists. Some states specifically allow a 96-hour emergency commitment if the patient is found to be seriously suicidal or homicidal, but the decision to commit involuntarily must be reviewed by a hearing officer, often within 24 hours after commitment. If after 96 hours it is decided that the patient needs further treatment, a civil commitment can be initiated by physicians but this too will usually be reviewed by a hearing officer within a short period of time. Because there have been abuses of the power to commit, many states have limited considerably the length of detainment and provided for continuing observation of the confined patient by a legal body such as the court or a hearing officer of the department of health.

Confidentiality

This is an area of growing importance, especially because of the recent passing of an act calling for Professional Standards Review Organizations (PSROs) which will consist primarily of specialists in each field of medicine who will participate in the peer review of records of other specialists. The implications of PSRO's in the mental health field in regard to confidentiality of patient information are significant. Records of patients will be available for review by other mental health workers, thus increasing the number of individuals who have access to this information. Consequently, there will be an increased possibility of personal data becoming public. Along with this, greater use of the computer in medical record-keeping has introduced another area for possible abuse of personal information. There is a growing need, therefore, to develop legal safeguards for protecting patients in the medical care system, as information regarding the mental health of an individual can be particularly damaging to his success in employment and to relationships outside the family.

Another issue concerning confidentiality of patient information arises when a psychiatrist is asked to reveal confidential information in a court proceeding. Many states have passed statutes which protect the privileged communication between physicians and patients, but federal courts have recently taken the position that privileged communication in court proceedings is no longer applicable in the general physician–patient relationship. They did however make an exception for testimony regarding mental illness.

In addition to these recent developments, it is important to note that the mental health worker has an obligation to treat information given to him by his patient as confidential. There also seems to be a trend toward letting patients see the information contained in their medical records.

The Patient's Rights While in the Hospital

In addition to the right to certain standards of psychiatric treatment, patients also have rights with regard to acceptance or rejection of certain medical procedures. Human experimentation has created an awareness of the right of patients to be fully informed of what is to be done to them and to give consent when possible. There is a special problem in regard to informed consent, in determining whether or not mentally ill or mentally retarded patients have the capacity to understand the nature of medical procedures. This issue is particularly important where procedures are considered clinically experimental. In fact, protection committees are now being established to safeguard the rights of the mentally ill and mentally retarded. Parents' informed consent must be obtained for treatment, whether experimental or not, of the mentally retarded or minors.

Testamentary Capacity

The patient's ability to make decisions involving his personal property or commitments is often called into question. Psychiatrists are frequently asked whether the patient has the ability to make a will; if he knows, for example, the value of his estate or those who are likely to be his heirs. Perhaps more to the point is whether the patient would be abnormally susceptible to persuasion by others. Similarly, the ability to make a contract or agreement—to purchase an expensive item or even to enter into marriage—requires an assessment of that patient's capacity to give consent relatively free from other influences. A patient suffering from serious delusions often acts under the influence of those delusions and consequently would be incapable of entering into a valid will or contract.

The Right to Terminate Treatment

The patient's right to terminate treatment in a mental institution depends upon whether he was voluntarily admitted or involuntarily committed. If he were voluntarily admitted to the institution, he has the right to terminate treatment whenever he wishes with few restrictions. Many of the states may require that he follow certain procedures for initiating termination of his treatment program in the hospital. The patient who has been involuntarily committed is in a different position. He is often denied the right to initiate termination of involuntary emergency hospitalization except for extraordinary reasons, although in some cases his efforts can result in legal intervention. Even the patient who voluntarily admits himself to a mental institution can, under certain conditions, be effectively denied the right to terminate treatment if during the course of his hospitalization he becomes seriously suicidal or homicidal. As with the other legal issues that affect the care of patients, states vary widely on their provisions for termination of treatment.

THE PSYCHIATRIST AS WITNESS

A psychiatrist is often called as a witness in civil or criminal trials involving patients. Although the psychiatrist's role is advisor to the court, he is often placed in a difficult position of being forced to respond to the sharply directed questions of the attorney but not given an opportunity to demonstrate fully the imprecision of psychiatric testimony. In addition to some of the problems involving confidentiality of patient information and testamentary capacity that have been briefly discussed, the psychiatrist is also likely to become involved in many other issues in his role as a witness.

The Insanity Defense

The determination of whether or not an offender can be held responsible for a criminal act is a difficult one for the court. Depending on the laws of the state in which the trial is being conducted, the psychiatrist might be asked to assess whether the offender had the cognitive capacity to distinguish between right and wrong when the crime occurred or to respond to the more complicated question of whether he was emotionally capable of exerting free will. There are a variety of tests used by the court to determine whether the offender should be held responsible for his acts. Each of these tests involves the expert opinion of the psychiatrist.

In addition to being called to respond to questions of criminal responsibility during a court proceeding, the psychiatrist is often asked to assist the prosecuting attorney and the judge to determine if the defendant is able to stand trial—if he is capable of understanding the allegations being brought against him and if he is able to participate in his own defense. Besides criminal cases, the psychiatrist may be asked to testify as to the existence of a mental illness caused by the negligence of another person (industrial or automobile accidents, *et cetera*).

Child Abuse

Mental health workers are sometimes confronted with the problems of child abuse. Most often, there will be some evidence of this, such as conspicuous bruise marks or signs of malnutrition. Other times it might be quite difficult to determine if in fact child abuse is occurring. What are the responsibilities of the mental health worker to the child? Is he legally obligated to intervene? If so, what course of action would be most appropriate when the mental health worker has a reasonable suspicion that child abuse is occurring? Is he held to a different degree of responsibility if the patient is the parent rather than the child? What are the responsibilities of a mental health worker when he is called as an expert witness to assess whether a child has been abused or if he is emotionally unstable and engaging in deception?

Sexual Deviancy

Various forms of sexual deviancy, homosexuality and sodomy, are classified as criminal behavior even between consenting adults. Mental health workers are often called to verify that an offender is deviant and to outline the possibilities for effective treatment. When sexual deviancy involves coercion or duress, as in acts against minors, the penalties might be quite severe. In such cases, the mental health worker could have a significant role as an advisor to the court in its decision as to appropriate sentencing. Also, he might have a voice in helping the parole authorities decide when conditional release would be appropriate. When the deviant behavior involves consenting adults, the mental health worker is often placed in a position of conflict. He may question the legitimacy of laws that outlaw sexual deviancy among consenting adults, yet still be asked to provide information on the psychiatric abnormality of such behavior which could be instrumental in the court's disposition of individual cases. Also the label of sexual deviancy often creates an inference that the offender engages in other acts that are injurious to others in the society.

Drug Addiction

The mental health worker is often asked to assist in deciding whether a defendant in a criminal case is a drug addict. The major difficulty in making such a determination concerns the definition of drug addiction. Should it be considered a "disease" and if so does this mean that the individual should become the responsibility of the medical profession for treatment or that of the criminal process for violating a specific law? A recent case brought before the U.S. Supreme Court resulted in that court deciding that drug addiction is not in and of itself a crime (Robinson vs California, 1962). By making this decision the court was in effect articulating the opinion that narcotic addiction is a disease and as such should not be subject to legal penalties but rather to therapeutic intervention. What responsibility does such a decision impose upon the mental health worker? There are instances where mental health workers are asked to testify about the effects drugs might have had on an individual's capacity to understand the nature of a criminal act. For example, a murderer might claim that he was under the influence of drugs to the extent that he was not aware of the implications of his actions. In many states such a declaration would be unlikely to excuse the offender completely from responsibility for his actions, but it might result in a lessening of the penalties.

Alcoholism

The issues surrounding alcoholism are similar to those in drug addiction. First, most courts view alcoholism as a disease similar to drug addiction and consequently not in and of itself a crime. The testimony of a mental health worker would be important in cases where chronic alcoholism, like drug addiction, was being presented as an excuse for criminal responsibility, or when an offender is required to undergo treatment for this condition and a mental health worker is asked to attest to the effectiveness of therapy in individual cases.

Divorce Proceedings

The mental health worker might at some time be called to testify about the capacity of a spouse to handle children. The decision as to which parent will get custody of the children is one of the most important issues in divorce proceedings. If one of the spouses, particularly the wife, is undergoing psychiatric treatment, the court might require that she prove she is mentally and emotionally capable of raising children. In states where privileged communications exist between a mental health worker, particularly a psychiatrist, and his patient, the psychiatrist is not required to respond to questions in court unless the privilege is waived by the patient. If the spouse requests that the psychiatrist testify that her mental condition will not affect her ability to care for children, she may waive the privilege of confidentiality of the physician-patient relationship. By waiving that privilege, though, the psychiatrist can be questioned on cross examination about other things that may have been disclosed during therapy. In those states where privileged communication between a psychiatrist and a patient is not honored, the psychiatrist can under certain circumstances be required to testify about his patient and produce his records.

THE PSYCHIATRIST AS DEFENDANT

A psychiatrist is susceptible to suits for malpractice. In the past, the test for malpractice was the standard of care rendered by a psychiatrist in comparison to the standards of the community in which he practiced. Today a new basis for comparison has emerged; the psychiatrist is measured against the standards of all psychiatrists rather than just those in his community.

Inadequate care. A bad outcome from a treatment program does not in itself mean that malpractice or negligence has occurred. It is important to show also that the psychiatrist acted unreasonably in the performance of his duties by omitting an essential therapy or administering treatment carelessly.

Inappropriate care. A psychiatrist may be accused of engaging in conduct inappropriate to the therapist-patient relationship. For example, psychiatrists have been accused of sexual assault on their patients. Included in this category would be the use of unique or possibly untried treatment methods which, if experimental, require informed consent by the patient. Some procedures might be so irregular they could not even be classified as experimental treatment. In such cases, a psychiatrist may be tried and convicted for recklessness and gross negligence. Abandonment or partial abandonment of the patient by the psychiatrist is another form of inappropriate care.

Institutional liability. Not only is the institution potentially liable for accidents which occur while the patient is hospitalized, but there also is a growing trend to impute liability to the institution for the level of care which it provides. To some extent this topic is entangled with the right to psychiatric treatment where courts are beginning to set standards for minimum care. But over and above this, the institution is becoming increasingly more susceptible to liability for inadequate and inappropriate care rendered by its mental health workers.

The patient–family–psychiatry–law interface is a complicated one. It is apparent from this discussion that there are many areas where these participants can come into conflict in the care of the mentally ill. Presented thus far has been a mere sketch of the issues that will be developed in depth around illustrative cases in the following chapters.

REFERENCES

Curran W J, Shapiro E D (1970): Law, Med Forensic Sci. Boston, Little Brown

Dawidoff D J (1966): The malpractice of psychiatrists. Duke Law J 696

Glueck S (1966): Law and Psychiatry: Cold War or Entente Cordiale. Baltimore, Johns Hopkins Press

King R (1972): The Drug Hang-Up: America's Fifty-Year Folly. New York, W W Norton

Kirbens S M (1968): Chronic alcohol addiction and criminal responsibility. 54 Am Bar Assn J 877

Morse H N (1967): The tort liability of psychiatrists. Baylor Law Rev 19:208

Musto D F (1973): The American Disease: Origins of Narcotic Control. New Haven, Yale University Press

Nason vs Superintendent of Bridgewater State Hospital, (1968) 353 Mass 604, 233 N E 2nd 908

Note (1967): Informed consent in medical malpractice. Calif Law Rev 55:1396

Plante M L (1968): Analysis of informed consent. Fordham Law Rev 36:639

Robinson vs California, (1962) 370 US 662

Rouse vs Cameron, (1966) 125 U S App D C 366, 373 S 2nd 451

Szasz T S (1969): When is inequality inequity? Georgetown Law Rev 57:734

Wyatt vs Stickney, (1972) 344 F Supp 373; 373 F Supp 387

3 DEFINITIONAL PROBLEMS IN PSYCHIATRY

Psychiatry stands in a unique position within the profession of medicine. Unlike internal medicine or surgery, many of the leading figures in psychiatry throughout the world and in various training programs or schools of thought here in the United States differ as to criteria for diagnosis and the course of treatment once diagnosis has been accomplished. A physician trained in internal medicine, when confronted by a man in his late sixties with severe chest pain radiating down the left arm, may suspect that the patient has a myocardial infarction (*i.e.*, "heart attack"). To corroborate his impression, he may administer an electrocardiogram (*i.e.*, "EKG"). If his diagnostic impression is correct, there are usually changes that clearly indicate damage to heart muscle. If fortunate enough to have a previous EKG for comparison, he can show that the wave patterns are recent, not old. Even if he doesn't, however, there are certain patterns characteristic of an occlusion of a coronary artery and these changes vary over the course of time to represent an active process involving damage to the patient's cardiac muscle. In addition, there are laboratory blood tests which also generally change at the time a patient has severe heart damage. The level of one enzyme, serum glutamic oxaloacetic transaminase (SGOT), rises steadily to the second or third day and then falls rapidly. There may also be an increase in the number of white blood cells for seven to ten days and an elevation of the erythrocyte sedimentation rate (ESR) that may last several weeks while the heart muscle heals. Thus a physician does not need to depend totally on his own clinical impression that a patient's chest pain is more than "heart burn" due to a regurgitation of acid from the stomach. He may corroborate his diagnosis of a heart attack by objective clinical and laboratory tests, in this instance, the electrocardiogram and serum enzyme values.

Consequently there is relatively little ambiguity as to the best course of treatment. A myocardial infarction is considered a medical emergency and requires intensive care during the acute phase. Not infrequently, death may occur early in the patient's course of therapy. Treatment measures include rest, adequate sedation, oxygen when indicated, a modification of diet so that during the first few days following the episode food is in a liquid or soft form and control of pain. As constipation may cause a problem with straining at stool, mild laxatives or stool softeners are given. If a complication arises such as congestive heart failure, shock or a cardiac arrhythmia, there are again specific diagnostic procedures to confirm the physician's clinical impression from a patient's history, and treatment is specific to the problem diagnosed.

The situation is not so simple when a psychiatric clinician is confronted with a patient with a psychiatric problem. The differences, in fact, are felt by some to be so great that they have seriously queried whether the medical model is truly appropriate for the evaluation and treatment of behavioral aberrations. There are several distinctive differences that merit discussion:

(1) **Psychiatric symptoms are universal.**

Unlike severe chest pain which generally points to a few specific diagnostic entities such as myocardial infarction or dissecting aortic aneurysm, most psychiatrists have experienced to some degree the symptoms that psychiatric patients present. There are a few psychiatric disorders in which the qualitative or quantitative variation from the norm is so extreme as to be deemed analogous to the severe chest pain of myocardial infarction. For example, the mild depression known by all with the loss of someone we have loved is quantitatively and qualitatively different from the syndrome of severe depression with involutional melancholia in mid-life. However, most of the symptoms patients come to therapy with are hard to distinguish from the conflicts, feelings and behaviors of individuals who do not seek psychotherapy.

The question, of course, arises among those of us who have a sociological bent as to whether it may not be more appropriate to study the variables which produce the treatment-seeking behavior rather than the factors that produce the symptoms. If after several years of marriage most people become a little depressed at the realization that all they had hoped for at the time of the initial commitment has not been accomplished, and it appears unlikely that it ever will, why do some just "grin and bear it," others divorce, and others seek psychiatric help? Comparably, as one individual reaches the sixth decade of his life and realizes that many of his ambitions to travel or to attain a certain amount of power, status, or wealth will not in all probability ever be actualized, and the idea of personal death, which once seemed so remote becomes more real, why does he come for help for the vague depression he feels, while another in similar circumstances does not?

Symptoms in fact are so prevalent that major studies have statistically demonstrated that it is more "normal" to have a symptom than not to have one. The Midtown Manhattan study (Srole *et al*, 1962) sampled 1660 adults between age 20 to 59 from an area of New York City with a population of about 175,000 (110,000 of whom were between the ages of 20 to 59). Their goal was to determine the mental health of the community members, most of whom had never been psychiatric patients. Subjects' mental health was rated on a scale of four levels—"well," "mild symptom formation," "moderate symptom function" and "impaired." The data used to determine the ratings was obtained through questionnaire-guided interviews by nonpsychiatrist interviewers. Psychiatrists then assessed the overall rating of mental health from the questionnaires. Only 19% were felt to be well. The remaining 81% were considered to have symptoms and a full 23% were rated markedly impaired to incapacitated.

Other population studies have confirmed the findings of Srole and his group in Manhattan. The Leightons (1963) undertook an extensive study of a rural area of Canada to evaluate the role of social disintegration in the genesis of mental illness. Again, the researchers studied an entire population and did not rely only on *treated* psychiatric illness. They found that only 20% of the men and 15% of the women showed no evidence of psychiatric disorder.

Another study of a "normal" population in Sweden by Essen–Möller (1956) found a somewhat greater proportion of the population to be free of psychiatric abnormalities (*i.e.*, 50% of the men and 42% of women).

It is clear from these studies that while the presence of symptoms may be a necessary reason for seeking psychiatric care, they are not sufficient cause. In fact, many people who never see a psychiatric clinician may be more sick than many of those who are treated.

(2) There are no unequivocal objective physical diagnostic signs or laboratory examinations in nonorganic psychiatric illness.

A physician may use the electrocardiogram and serum enzyme values to confirm his diagnostic impression that a patient has had a myocardial infarction, but there are no clear-cut tests for a psychotic depression or schizophrenia, nor for the so-called neuroses or character disorders. This is, of course, not true for the organic psychiatric disorders occurring in hyperthyroidism or Huntington's Chorea. In both these disorders there are mental changes labeled "psychoses" by most psychiatric clinicians, and objective physical or biochemical changes. The psychiatric and physical symptoms are the result of an underlying physical disease process. In hyperthyroidism there is excess activity of the thyroid gland; physical signs include increased heart rate or protuberance of the eyes (exopthalmos). In addition, the serum protein bound iodine is elevated. In Huntington's chorea, the behavioral disorder is usually accompanied by abnormal bodily movements such as chorea or athetosis. The disorder characteristically has its onset at about age 35 and one-half of the members of a patient's family show a similar disorder.

The diagnosis of nonorganic psychiatric illness, even severe psychosis, is not so easily confirmed. What may be labeled schizophrenia in one country may be called manic–depressive illness in another (Lieb and Slaby, 1975). There is a growing body of literature implicating genetic factors (Kallman, 1953; Slater, 1953, Fieve, 1973, Rosenthal, 1973) and metabolic factors (Schildkraut, 1965, 1970; Bunney & Davis, 1965) in the major psychiatric disorders. As yet, however, no standardized laboratory tests have been developed which might serve to confirm a clinical diagnosis.

Even if it were possible to confirm a diagnosis, however, this would not necessarily exculpate a person from socially unacceptable conduct. An individual may still be fully aware of the implications of his action despite the presence of a psychiatric illness.

(3) Psychiatrists, unlike their medical colleagues, often disagree on the definition of mental illness.

It would be difficult to find many physicians who would disagree that a myocardial infarction is an illness and that it requires treatment. This is not the case in dealing with behavioral aberrations. Lawyers concerned with precision of definition are often dismayed at the difficulties psychiatrists have in deciding whether a patient is schizophrenic or manic-depressive, or that psychiatrists may even disagree as to whether an individual's markedly aberrant behavior represents a severe psychotic disorder or a normal response to a "crazy" world.

This viewpoint that aberrant behavior is actually within the range of normal responses is exemplified in the writings of Thomas Szasz (1957, 1960, 1964). Szasz raises the question as to whether there is such a thing as mental illness and decides in favor of its nonexistence. He feels that psychiatric clinicians tend to see problems of living as disturbances which have analogs in the medical disease model. In fact, as he points out, many contemporary physicians and scientists feel that ultimately a neurological defect, albeit subtle, may be found some day to explain any behavioral disturbances. Szasz feels that for the sake of clarity people who speak of mental illness meaning brain disease should call it that. However, he feels that mental illness is usually diagnosed when an individual's behavior deviates from certain legal, psychosocial or ethical norms and that these deviations are expected to be correctable by medical action. Since these are essentially problems in human living that have been defined as illness by nonmedical criteria, Szasz feels it is absurd to believe that medical treatment will help to prevent their occurrence.

Obviously Szasz' ideas about the determination and treatment of mental illness represent a radical extreme. Nevertheless, his ideas have an important heuristic function especially in the assessment of behavior that is contrary to legal norms.

When determination of who is ill or not ill is relatively subjective or at least not agreed upon by those in the profession assigned this task, the implications become infinitely more difficult to unravel.

(4) The presence of a "symptom" does not imply mental illness, nor does a complex of symptoms per se lessen an individual's responsibility for his actions.

This is perhaps no more graphically illustrated than in the case of suicide. Suicide may be a symptom of a psychotic depression or schizophrenia, but while some feel that one must be "crazy" to want to take one's own life there are several instances in which an individual who attempts or successfully accomplishes suicide may be quite sane. A person in extreme pain from an incurable cancer may quite rationally decide to take his own life. A comparable line of reasoning suggests that homicide, which some may also argue is so cruel that a person has to be "insane" to commit it, may also be a rational decision. Just as certain behavior, even homicide or suicide, is not *prima facie* evidence of mental illness, the fact that a patient is unequivocally schizophrenic does not always mean that he is not responsible for his actions. A person may have a disorganization of his thought processes but still be responsible for his actions in a given situation. Each situation must be examined individually to see how much the individual involved should be considered responsible for his actions.

(5) There is disagreement among psychiatrists as to the treatment of choice for many psychiatric illnesses.

The choice of treatment in psychiatry is usually not as certain as in other specialties of medicine. If a person has a myocardial infarction he would be treated by most physicians as outlined in the beginning of this chapter. If he has childhood-onset diabetes, he would be treated with insulin and regulation of diet and exercise. If hypothyroid, he would be given a thyroid preparation. The only really analogous psychiatric situation would be the treatment of manic-depressive illness with lithium carbonate. Patients with schizophrenia may be treated with a variety of approaches from major tranquilizers to psychoanalytically oriented psychotherapy.

Dispute over therapeutic approaches generates even greater confusion for those involved in the assessment and treatment of individuals considered "sociopathic."

This ambiguity bewilders trainees in the mental health professions and lawyers seeking precision in diagnostic evaluations and consensually validated treatment recommendations.

Such issues have made it difficult to ascertain exactly what role mental health professionals should play in the legal process. If a psychiatrist employs a medical model in the evaluation of a patient for the defense attorney, the prosecuting lawyer may find a psychiatrist who, using a sociological concept for viewing behavior, may give an entirely different interpretation of a patient's condition. Testimony involving the use of psychodiagnostic tests such as the Rorschach may raise the issue of the tests' validity. At this point, with rare exceptions, there are no simple solutions. Much of the criticism of the state of contemporary psychiatry is valid. While there are some objective definitions of mental illness and some specific treatments, there are still many improvements to be made. The definition of genetic factors in manic–depressive illness, the phenomonological characteristics of unipolar and bipolar depression, and the discovery of the efficacy of lithium carbonate in the treatment of manic–depressive illness represent much needed advances on which future achievements will hopefully be modelled.

There are a few general guidelines which we may use in our approach to the evaluation of a patient's behavior when a legal question is raised. Among these is the fact that although a condition may be defined as mental illness by any given definition, the individual is not dysfunctional in all areas. Much like a medical patient who may be confined to bed rest with all active employment prohibited, a psychiatric patient may need a few months to recompensate in a hospital following a psychological disintegration. But despite the restriction on activity, he may still be able to make out a will or understand the nature of a contract. Evaluation of his ability to perform must be made specifically for the task that is required. He may be diagnosed as schizophrenic but still be aware of the extent of his property and who his heirs are. Furthermore, the criteria for involuntary confinement to a hospital should be strictly defined. The simplest ethical solution would be to limit involuntary confinement totally to those individuals who are severely psychotic or when there is danger that an individual will harm himself or others.

In the following two sections legal–psychiatric problems confronting the mental health professional in his daily work will be discussed. These chapters focus on situations in which the psychiatric clinician may be called upon to make decisions that may or may not require an interaction with the legal system. Illustrative case examples of the most typical problems will be presented. The specific questions that they raise will be clearly articulated and the information that must be sought to answer these will be presented. In all instances, we will take the rather traditional approach that there is indeed something called mental illness. In the psychoses, and in particular manic–depressive psychosis, there is reasonable approximation of the medical model of illness and a medical approach to treatment. In cases such as the neuroses and character disorders which are vaguer entities, the difficulties in assessment are considerably greater. If what is really involved is a "problem of living," the behavior in question should be treated as such but a psychiatric clinician may still be able to offer valuable recommendations in management, as in the case of divorce proceedings. Some psychiatric entities are so vaguely defined and treatment so ambiguous that they are confusing to all concerned.

It is inevitable that the reader may disagree with some of our ideas. For instance, sociopathy is felt by many to be a personality or character disorder. Yet to dismiss criminal acts as products of mental illness because the offenders are "sociopathic" —the victims of an unfavorable early childhood environment or an undesirable genetic predisposition that has molded them into individuals without any conscious choice—would be to take a deterministic view of behavior that carried *reductio ad absurdem* would remove all individual responsibility for criminal action. This is not a posture we espouse. Sociopathy may be a descriptive term for a form of behavior in which individuals seem to have neither conscience nor concern for societal rules or penalties, but it does not mean such individuals are mentally ill.

Perhaps some day the term "sociopathy" will be deleted from the classification of the American Psychiatric Association with much of the same controversy that the elimination of the diagnosis of "homosexuality" has created. Homosexuality, like sociopathy, describes a behavior, in this case sexual interests, attraction, or relations with a member of the same sex. It does not imply lack of responsibility for action any more than heterosexuality does, nor does it exculpate a person from responsibility for his actions. A number of variants of heterosexual and homosexual behavior may be symptomatic of mental illness just as alterations in food appetites may be. So, too, some criminal or sociopathic behavior may be the signs of a person becoming mentally ill. But this does not mean that all or even the majority of those accused of crimes are becoming mentally ill. The perennial existence of social illness does not justify abdication of personal responsibility.

The broader issues of the psychiatric clinician's responsibility to the patient, the responsibility he has to the greater society and the appropriate level of interest of the mental health professional in the patient–law interface will be discussed in the final three chapters.

REFERENCES

Bunney WE, Davis JM (1965): Norepinephrine in depressive reactions: A review. Arch Gen Psychiatry 13:483

Essen-Möller E (1956): Individual traits and morbidity in a Swedish rural population. Acta Psychiat Scand (Suppl) 100

Kallmann FJ (1953): Heredity in Health and Mental Disorder. New York, W W Norton

Leighton DC, Harding JS, Macklin DB, Macmillan AM, Leighton AH (1963): The Character of Danger. New York, Basic Books

Lieb J, Slaby AE (1975): Integrated Psychiatric Treatment. New York, Harper & Row

Schildkraut JJ (1965): The catecholamine hypothesis of affective disorders: A review of supporting evidence. Am J Psychiatry 122:509

Schildkraut JJ (1970): Neuropsychopharmacology and the Affective Disorders. Boston, Little Brown

Slater, E (1953): Psychotic and neurotic illnesses in twins, Medical Research Council (Special Report Series). London, No 278

Srole, L, Langner, TS, Michael, ST, Opler, MK, Rennie TAC (1962): Mental Health in the Metropolis. New York, McGraw-Hill

Szasz TS (1957): The problem of psychiatric nosology: A contribution to a situational analysis of psychiatric operations. Am J Psychiatry 114:405–413

Szasz TS (1960): The myth of mental illness. Am Psychol 15:113–118

Szasz TS (1964): The Myth of Mental Illness. New York, Harper & Row

PART **2**

THE RIGHTS
OF **THE PATIENT**

4 THE RIGHT TO PSYCHIATRIC TREATMENT

Admissions to the psychiatric care system fall into two general groups. One group is on a voluntary basis and the other involuntary. Truly involuntary admissions through court commitment involve a distinct minority of cases. Usually, in an instance where an individual is considerably disturbed, he may be persuaded by a spouse, another relative or a friend to admit himself voluntarily to a psychiatric hospital for observation and treatment. There remain, however, a number of instances where patients either have caused sufficient disturbance or have refused despite gross psychopathological behavior to admit themselves so that their involuntary commitment becomes necessary. Usually one finds a group of patients like this in any large state mental hospital. Some may in fact have been brought to court but prior to trial were found unable to participate in their own defense and were committed to a mental hospital pending such time when they would be able to do so.

Instances have been brought to light where patients have stayed in large hospitals with staffs so small they are capable of providing only custodial care and little active treatment. In such a circumstance one may well imagine a situation in which a psychotic individual quite innocent of a crime could be implicated by circumstantial evidence. While he might have been able to exonerate himself if he were not psychiatrically ill, in his state of psychosis he would have been unable to participate in his own defense and therefore was committed to a state mental hospital to come to trial at a later date. But if he is not given active treatment with the hope that he might recover to a sufficient degree to defend himself, he may remain incarcerated for a longer period than if he had been found guilty of a minor crime and imprisoned for a limited period.

There are other issues to be considered in defining psychiatric treatment from the standpoint of right to treatment. These include both the qualitative and quantitative aspects of the therapy process. What is high quality psychiatric care and how much should be given to be considered an adequate amount? Or in cases where a patient doesn't respond, what is considered a "fair trial" of a given treatment? Good psychiatric care is not so easily defined as good medical care. There are many approaches, many potentially equally effective. Psychiatry is in great need of cost-effectiveness studies. Does long-term psychoanalysis really cause any objective changes which can be considered better than those of another form of treatment or better than no treatment at all, or are its effects so subjective that a patient's or clinician's own philosophical or theoretical position determines how the end result of a treatment process is viewed? And even if a treatment is relatively more effective, does its additional cost merit its use over another that is nearly as effective but considerably less expensive?

Finally a review of the factors which must be borne in mind when examining a patient's "right to treatment" should also include an examination of a patient's right not to be treated. If a Christian Scientist who is psychotic refuses treatment with a phenothiazine, may a physician still give him the needed treatment? And, if a patient is psychotic and needs psychopharmacotherapy, can his Christian Science relatives legally prevent the treatment?

HYPOTHETICAL CASE ILLUSTRATION: R.T., a 38-year-old black, Baptist, divorced, construction worker, two months following the death of his mother, began to hear her voice at night telling him to be "good" and "clean up vice." At first he kept these thoughts to himself but soon these voices began to occur during the day and told him that "homosexuals and other sex perverts" who worked with him were after his "body." He became increasingly suspicious and quick to pick fights over such petty instances as being bumped accidentally by a fellow employee. After several complaints by his fellow workers about his changed, argumentative and erratic behavior, his foreman called him in and asked what caused him to act this way. Blandly he stated that there was a conspiracy of "sexual perverts" who were trying to corrupt him and use his "body" for illicit purposes. He said his mother told him so from her place in heaven. When the foreman reacted with alarm, R.T. said it was apparent he was also part of the plot and angrily quit.

The area of the city where he had been working had several unisex shops. One of these had mannequins of ambiguous sexual identity with various wigs cut in popular mod styles. After staring at them, he picked up several garbage cans and threw them, one at a time, at the window, smashing the glass and hitting people seated in the waiting room. When police rushed to stop him, he fought them off stating "God" told him to put an end to all "modern sex and corruption."

The patient was jailed and while awaiting trial, the prosecuting attorney for the state met with the patient's lawyer from the public defender service and concurred that R.T. was incapable of standing trial. The patient was then sent to a large state mental hospital in the city in which he lived. Two years later, a public defender attorney attached to the hospital found that the patient was still there and remained delusional. Knowing of the minimal staffing in the hospital, the attorney queried whether he was being actively treated as he had not recovered and did not therefore have the opportunity to return to trial either to be found guilty or set free.

DISCUSSION

The primary issue in this hypothetical example concerns the right to treatment for those involuntarily hospitalized. The importance of the right to treatment is particularly poignant in this case since the reputed offender had not even been convicted of a crime. He was required, instead, to undergo involuntary admission for the purpose of treatment prior to defending himself in a court trial. Many states have statutes which require periodic examination of those involuntarily committed. Patients who have been involuntarily hospitalized should not be coerced to remain in confinement when the medical and statutory qualifications no longer require hospitalization. At least 22 states require such periodic examinations, mandatory every six months or once a year; in some states frequency is not specified.

The concept of the right to treatment originating in statutes that require periodic examination and judicial review of those involuntarily committed is a relatively recent development. It received its primary impetus from a late 1960 case in the District of Columbia where the appeals court decided that according to the District of Columbia code there was a statutory right to treatment (Rouse vs Cameron, 1966). On the basis of this decision, a District of Columbia court confronted with the issue of adequacy of treatment must decide not only whether the treatment—in particular periodic examinations, staffing capacities and physical facilities of the hospital—meets at least minimum professional standards, but in addition whether the treatment is appropriate for the patient's individual requirements.

The District of Columbia statute and court case, therefore, enunciated an important general principle regarding patients' rights to treatment. In effect, this principle states that when a patient is hospitalized involuntarily, there is an obligation to provide the treatment which serves the ends for which the individual is hospitalized. If this treatment is not provided, then the patient could be either transferred, released or even awarded damages for the period of commitment.

Other similar cases were brought to trial in behalf of patients who were not receiving any treatment. In the Massachusetts case, the court found that the mental hospital involved was grossly understaffed and that the patient was not receiving acceptable treatment (Nason vs Bridgewater, 1968). These cases have certainly had an important role in highlighting the issues surrounding the right to treatment, but it is questionable whether they resulted in any major improvement in the treatment of mental patients in most state institutions. Only a few other jurisdictions have in fact followed the line of reasoning outlined in the District of Columbia case and recognized the right to treatment as a legal doctrine.

The most significant advance in *expanding* the doctrine of the right to treatment was made in the early 1970s with a case involving a large number of patients suing the mental health commissioner of Alabama for the inadequacy of care at a state institution. (Wyatt vs Stickney, 1972). The federal district court in Alabama, upon reviewing the staff and facilities at this state institution, held that persons involuntarily confined in institutions for the mentally retarded and mentally ill have a Constitutional right to both adequate treatment and living conditions. Although the case is presently being appealed to a higher court, the federal district court that decided in favor of the patients established what it considered judicially enforceable standards which can be used to measure adequate treatment. The minimum standards include not only medical requirements such as minimum staff standards, individualized evaluations of residents, and treatment plans and programs, but also detailed physical standards and nutritional requirements, the establishment of a Human Rights Committee at all institutions, the insurance of a humane psychological environment and even the requirement that patients be compensated for work accomplished while in the mental facility. If this decision is upheld, it will be a landmark, for it goes beyond the earlier right to treatment case in the District of Columbia by holding that an entire state mental health system was Constitutionally inadequate and that judicially enforceable standards for health care in mental facilities are required.

Some courts in other jurisdictions have recently taken the position that there is no Constitutional right to treatment (Burnham vs Georgia, 1973), but the Alabama case will likely begin a major trend toward judicial decisions in favor of the right to treatment in mental facilities. This observation is supported by the decision in a Florida case in 1972 where a patient, hospitalized for many years in a state facility without adequate treatment, was awarded damages of $38,000 against a staff psychiatrist and the superintendent of a state hospital (Donaldson vs O'Connor).*

The Constitutional basis for the right to treatment is found in two provisions of the Eighth and Fourteenth Amendments of the Constitution. The Eighth Amendment deals with the issue of cruel and unusual punishment. In a decision in 1968, the Supreme Court precluded punishment for involuntary behavior stemming from mental illness or chronic drug addiction. According to the court, sickness should not be treated as though it were a criminal offense in itself. With this decision in mind, the argument logically follows that commitment without treatment of the mentally ill violates the Eighth Amendment.

The two provisions of the Fourteenth Amendment are those dealing with due process or fundamental fairness and equal protection of laws. According to the doctrine of "fundamental fairness," there must be a reasonable relationship between the nature and duration of confinement of an individual and the purpose of that commitment. The equal protection of laws provision prohibits denying any citizen equal protection of the laws. This means in effect that classifying certain persons as mentally ill or handicapped and then depriving them of their personal liberty is reasonable only if it means that treatment will be provided. The system of classification would be unreasonable if the mentally handicapped were denied treatment because then only they would be selected for "preventive detention" while other individuals who are potentially "dangerous" but who have not actually committed criminal acts are free from confinement.

Right to treatment cases are being introduced in various courts throughout the country; some courts have already upheld the principle that mental patients and the mentally retarded do have a right to treatment. The importance of these cases cannot be underestimated since they not only will involve major restructuring and alterations of the care of mental patients, but will also by introducing the concept of judicially enforced standards be likely to have effects throughout the medical care system.

In addition to the major issue regarding the right to treatment, other questions are also raised by this hypothetical case.

1) Is there a right to refuse treatment? The important decisions in the past have focused on the commitment process with little interest in what happens after the patient is hospitalized. The right to treatment cases have introduced the issue of whether a patient has a right to refuse treatment once committed. In 1971 the Second Circuit Court of Appeals in an important case—the Winters case (Winters

See Addendum, p. 159.

vs Miller, 1971)—held that mental patients have a Constitutional right to refuse medication—particularly, as in this case—on religious grounds. The case was appealed to the Supreme Court of the United States, but that court in December 1971 said that it would let the Second Circuit Court's decision stand.

2) Is there a right to treatment for others besides the mentally ill? The Supreme Court decision in the *Robinson* case (Robinson vs California, 1972) in the early 1960s was of major significance because essentially it disputed the appropriateness of punishment for involuntary behavior. In this case the court considered drug addiction a sickness and felt it inappropriate to subject the addict to the criminal process for his condition. Subsequent cases relying on this Supreme Court decision —that a person is not to be convicted of a crime for behavior that he cannot control —overruled the traditional notion of drunkenness as a crime in itself. (Driver vs Hinnant, 1966; Easter vs District of Columbia, 1966). In the late 1960s, the President's U.S. Crime Commission recommended substituting treatment programs for rehabilitation of alcoholics in place of the criminal process. As a result of the growing support for viewing alcoholism as a sickness, in 1968 Congress enacted the District of Columbia Alcoholic Rehabilitation Act which in essence substitutes comprehensive treatment programs for criminal sanctions in the handling of alcoholics.

During that same year a case involving an alcoholic was brought before the Supreme Court of the United States. (Powell vs Texas, 1968). The Supreme Court recognized that in the case of alcoholics whose intoxication is involuntary (as with chronic alcoholics), conviction is precluded by the Eighth Amendment; but the Court did not provide immunity from criminal action from the crime of public drunkenness for all alcoholics. The distinction, therefore, is not that alcoholism in general should deserve special treatment in the legal system but rather that chronic alcoholism, or that which is involuntary because the person has lost the selfcontrol with respect to intoxicating beverages, must be handled in a treatment setting. The principle then that the Supreme Court upheld from the earlier Robinson case is that an individual should not be subject to criminal penalties for being in a condition (such as chronic alcoholism or drug addiction) that he has become powerless to change.

The earlier cases which overturned convictions of alcoholics for the offense of public drunkenness still allow *chronic* alcoholics to be appropriately detained for treatment and rehabilitation as long as they are not characterized as criminals. By qualifying the involuntary commitment of chronic alcoholics in this manner, these courts condone confinement only when alcoholics can be considered a "menace to society" and for diagnosis and treatment. The District of Columbia Alcoholic Rehabilitation Act, which no longer views public intoxication as a criminal offense, explicitly requires that the chronic alcoholic be provided with adequate medical, psychiatric and rehabilitative treatment: ". . . that a chronic alcoholic is a sick person who needs, is entitled to, and shall be provided appropriate medical, psychiatric, institutional, advisory and rehabilitative treatment services of the highest caliber for his illness." (District of Columbia Alcoholic Rehabilitation Act, 1968).

In addition to the involuntary commitment of alcoholics, many states authorize similar confinement of drug addicts. As with alcoholism, right to treatment has assumed prominence so that confinement of drug addicts can only be condoned where treatment and rehabilitation are appropriately provided. In addition to chronic alcoholics and drug addicts, sexual psychopaths are also subject to involuntary commitment. In the past, commitment to a mental institution did not necessarily mean that the sexual psychopath would receive treatment and rehabilitative services. The right to treatment for these patients is only beginning to emerge. Again, the District of Columbia has taken the lead. A case in the late 1960s clearly stated that the confinement of sexual psychopaths, according to the District of Columbia statute, is justified only if treatment is provided (Millard vs Cameron, 1966). Courts in other jurisdictions of the country are beginning to extend the "right to treatment" to the sexual psychopath.

3) What are the implications of the "right to treatment" in terms of psychiatric practice? Early in the development of the right to treatment doctrine, its underlying purpose was to make sure public institutions would meet certain minimum quantitative standards for staffing and for physical facilities so that those involuntarily committed would be given appropriate treatment. With the adjudication of the cases discussed in this section, the role of the court has expanded considerably. Judicially enforced standards involve not only staffing patterns and facilities, but also physician visits, treatment plans and programs, and the evaluation of the quality of care provided by psychiatric residents. There has been an intrusion, therefore, into the very practice of psychiatry that could conceivably significantly influence the effectiveness and efficiency of psychiatric care. Assessing the effectiveness of treatment may require the use of random clinical trials much as have been used in traditional internal medicine to determine if in fact conventional treatment methods such as psychotherapy and psychoanalysis do have an advantage, not only over medication, but over no treatment at all.

The use of random clinical trials in internal medicine resulted in questioning the effectiveness of traditional practices such as coronary care units and oral diabetic agents. By comparing groups receiving different treatments, the random clinical trial is the major technique available for determining if a certain diagnostic or therapeutic procedure effectively serves the ends for which it was developed and ameliorates the natural history of a disease. The right to treatment doctrine as it is now articulated by the courts does not limit its concerns to staff and physical facilities but also concerns itself with treatment plans and programs which might ultimately include a determination of the quality of care being provided in institutions. The demands of the right to treatment doctrine, therefore, are far-reaching, including not only that treatment be provided to those involuntarily committed, but also that the nature of the treatment and its potential effectiveness be evaluated. This latter concern as it develops could have a major effect on the practice of psychiatry in the very near future. In this regard, however, physicians must be cautious or the legal profession will dictate standards of medical practice. More simply stated, there is evidently an increasing encroachment by the legal profession into the field of medicine. It is unclear whether in the final analysis this will have a salutory or detrimental effect on medical practice.

4) Has the right to treatment doctrine had any effect on other patient rights? Along with the right to treatment, there has been an examination of other rights of the mentally ill including the right to be compensated for their work in the hospital, and the right to an education which is particularly important to the mentally and socially handicapped child. Patients in many large state mental institutions are accustomed to performing various menial tasks such as kitchen work, waiting on tables, housekeeping and even patient care. In the past, such labors have gone unrewarded, but recently steps have been taken to end this institutional peonage. Some states have bills pending to abolish the use of patients

without compensation, and suits are being brought to prevent such peonage on the basis of the Thirteenth Amendment of the Constitution which forbids involuntary servitude except for punishment of convicted criminals.

One of the arguments for uncompensated labor has been that such tasks are part of the therapy and therefore do not require compensation. The position being taken by those challenging the use of patients in this manner is that even if the involuntary or coerced work is therapeutic, it still violates the prohibition set forth in the Thirteenth Amendment. Perhaps even more significant is the argument against making patients do distasteful hospital tasks as part of a therapeutic program.

REFERENCES

Bazelon J D L (1969): Implementing the right to treatment. University Chicago Law Rev 36:742

Birnbaum M (1968): Rationale for the right. Georgetown Law J 57:752

Brakel SJ, Rock RS (1971): The Mentally Disabled and the Law. Chicago, University of Chicago Press

Burnham vs State of Georgia, (1973) (Civ Action No 16385, N D Ga)

District of Columbia Code Annotated, (1967) Section 21–526 states that "a person hospitalized in a public hospital for mental illness shall during his hospitalization be entitled to medical and psychiatric care and treatment."

District of Columbia Alcoholic Rehabilitation Act (1968): Pub Law No 90–452, 82 Stat 618

Donaldson vs O'Connor, (1973) (Civ Action No 1693 N D Fla)

Driver vs Hinnant, (1966) 356 F 2d 761 (4th Cir)

Easter vs District of Columbia, (1966) 124 US App DC 33, 361 F 2d 50 (En Banc)

Ennis B J (1972): Prisoners of Psychiatry—Mental Patients, Psychiatrists and the Law. New York, Harcourt, Brace and Jovanovich

Halpern CR (1968): A practicing lawyer views the right to treatment. Georgetown Law J 57:782

Hutt PB, Merrill RA (1968): Criminal responsibility and the right to treatment for intoxication and alcoholism. Georgetown Law J 57:835

Mental Health Law Project (1973): Basic Rights of the Mentally Handicapped. Published by the Mental Health Law Project, Washington, D C

Millard vs Cameron, (1966) 373 F 2d 468, (D C Cir)

Nason vs Bridgewater, (1968) 233 NE 2d 908

Note (1967): Civil restraint, mental illness and the right to treatment. Yale Law J 77:87

Powell vs Texas, (1968) 392 US 514

President's Commission on Law Enforcement and Administration of Justice: Task Force Report (1967): Drunkenness. 1–6

Robinson vs California, (1972) 370 U S 660

Rouse vs Cameron, (1966) 373 F 2d 451

Weintraub FJ, Abeson A (1972): Appropriate education for all handicapped children: A growing issue. Syracuse Law Rev 24:15

Winters vs Miller, (1971) 446 F 2d 65

Wyatt vs Stickney, (1972) 344 F Supp 373 and 344 F Supp 387 (MD Ala)

CERTIFICATION
5 AND COMMITMENT
PROCEDURES

Under many circumstances a psychiatrically ill individual admits himself voluntarily to a mental hospital or psychiatric ward of a general hospital; a prospective patient enters the treatment situation on his own free will and usually signs a paper stating that he is voluntarily seeking psychiatric treatment.

In a number of situations, however, an individual may not consciously want psychiatric help or may be so psychotic that he is unaware that he is ill. If the physician who examines him or others are concerned that he may bring serious harm to himself and decide that he should be hospitalized, they may attempt to have him involuntarily committed to a psychiatric treatment facility. This means that he is committed for treatment without his consent and in some circumstances this may involve physical coercion. State laws vary as to how patients who do not willingly consent to treatment but are significantly psychiatrically ill may be committed to mental institutions. These laws have been designed to protect individuals who are not mentally ill from being detained in mental hospitals against their will for political, economic, family or other nonmedical reasons.

The first and easiest route for involuntary commitment is by medical certification. This relatively nontraumatic procedure usually involves examination by one or more physicians. If the patient is considered dangerous to himself or to others, a printed form is completed by one or possibly two licensed physicians— some states require that at least one physician be a psychiatrist—giving the results of the examination and the justification for involuntary hospitalization. In other instances, a more formal legal proceeding may take place and the patient is committed by the court. Both of these procedures, as well as an elaboration of criteria for medical certification, will be discussed in greater detail at the end of this chapter.

HYPOTHETICAL CASE EXAMPLE C.P. is a 23-year-old white, single, graduate student at a private eastern university who, following the ingestion of an unknown drug given to him by a person he met in a city park, began to feel unreal and apart from himself. At times he felt he observed himself as a stranger from afar. He looked dazed and sounded vaguely incoherent when his girlfriend met him one hour after he took the unknown drug. She took him to a local storefront crisis intervention center where he stayed for four hours but remained somewhat dazed and appeared distant to those who spoke to him. When it was suggested that he go to the emergency room of a general hospital, he resisted saying he was doing his "own thing." Scared that something was seriously wrong with C.P., three of the volunteers at the crisis center with the aid of his girlfriend got him into a car and took him to the emergency room.

When they arrived they found that the psychiatrist on duty was inundated with several severely psychotic, belligerent patients. The psychiatrist, therefore, asked a psychiatric nurse working with him to interview the patient. She did so and felt uneasy because the patient seemed so distant and vague and resistant to voluntary hospitalization. She reported to the emergency room psychiatrist that she felt that the patient might be undergoing a schizophrenic break and that he might "hurt himself or someone else." The psychiatrist hearing her evaluation concurred that the patient needed hospitalization but because he was busy did not examine the patient himself; instead he filled out a medical certification with information from the nurse. The patient continued to refuse hospitalization and when the ambulance attendants came to take him to the local state hospital, he forcibly resisted but was successfully overpowered.

The next day he was entirely back to normal and called his lawyer and personal physician to seek his release from the hospital. As the attending psychiatrist at the state hospital found his mental state to be within normal limits and felt that there was no need for further hospitalization, he was released without requiring any effort on the part of his lawyer or personal physician.

DISCUSSION

This case illustrates strikingly the many intricate features of involuntary admission to a mental facility. From the description of the patient, it appeared that he presented with the required characteristics for *emergency hospitalization* or detention. At least 40 states have statutes which provide for emergency detention where formal application has been made by a law enforcement or health officer; over a fourth of these states require that approval for detention be obtained from a judge, county clerk or possibly prosecuting attorney. Under some conditions, a local board of health or county commissioners may be empowered with the right to approve an emergency detention. In the remaining states judicial approval is not required but a medical certificate must be completed by a psychiatrist or other physician which states that he has examined the patient and concludes that he should be admitted. Some states require that only one physician examine the patient at the time that the certificate is made out, but others require the signature of two physicians. In addition to examination by those certifying mental illness, some states also require that the patient be examined by a physician at the institution where he is about to be admitted. Should this physician disagree with the diagnosis, the patient would have to be released immediately.

In C.P.'s case, one could justify emergency hospitalization on the basis of the criterion that the patient appeared to be in a state of present danger to himself or others. The fact, that the psychiatrist did not examine the patient but relied on the evaluation of the psychiatric nurse calls into serious question the validity of this involuntary hospitalization. Most states require that accompanying the application for admission, there be at least one certificate that personal examination has been made of the patient by a physician and was found to be sufficiently mentally ill as to require hospitalization.

Although this will be discussed in greater depth in a subsequent chapter, one interesting feature of the emergency hospitalization statutes is that they allow detainment in a mental health institution only until proper legal steps are taken for additional hospitalization. Most statutes contain special provisions which specifically limit the length of time that a patient may be detained. This may be anywhere from 24 hours in a few of the states to 30 days in many states and even 60 days in at least one. The justification for limiting detention is that hospitalization under emergency circumstances is intended primarily as a means of controlling an immediate threat. If the patient is to be detained further, the statutes often require that a court be notified and a hearing conducted.

In addition to detention through emergency hospitalization, there is also another form of commitment which is of a temporary or determinate nature, that is, *temporary* or *observational hospitalization.* This form of commitment is a relatively recent device primarily for the purpose of diagnosing a case and possibly providing short-term treatment. This type of commitment does not require a clear emergency such as emergency hospitalization does but rather is used for prompt and effective observation of a patient without the time delays that accompany more formal commitment procedures. Nearly 30 states have enacted separate procedures for temporary or observational hospitalization. Such hospitalization may be independent from the more formal involuntary hospitalization procedures, in which case there is no requirement for a formal application for reporting evidence of the need for extended hospitalization. Other states may require applications and certification procedures as well as a hearing before a judicial officer.

Temporary or observational hospitalization may also be used in connection with formal judicial hospitalization. A judge may adjourn a hearing on involuntary commitment and require that the patient be hospitalized for a specific period of time before a final decision is made on long-term or indeterminate commitment. Several states, including New York and California, require that temporary observation precede the decision to commit the patient for an indeterminate period of time. This decision in many states must also be made by a judge or court authority.

The emergency and temporary observational hospitalization procedures are for a determinate period of time. In contrast, formal commitment procedures exist which involve confinement for an indeterminate period after either a judicial hearing or medical certification. Formal commitment, particularly before a judge, is the most common form of involuntary hospitalization, though there appears to be a significant trend away from judicial commitment. Now, 40 states allow for some form of judicial hospitalization. This procedure requires that a judge or possibly a jury determine whether a person is mentally ill to the extent that hospitalization is necessary. Nearly all of the states have statutes that require that a prehearing medical examination be conducted by a physician who will attest to examining the patient and finding him mentally ill and in need of commitment. The elements of the judicial commitment consist of a petition or an application, a hearing before a judge or jury, and a final determination of whether the patient should be hospitalized. The petition includes an application which in many states may be signed by any citizen, though some states allow only specific persons such as spouses, relatives, friends and physicians the right to file an application for commitment of a patient. A medical certificate required by statute often accompanies the petition. In many states, the court is then required to give notice to the patient that the petition has been filed. Notice is given so that the patient can have an opportunity with the assistance of legal counsel to prepare for the hearing in the event that he wishes to contest it. The hearing is often held in a probate court or in a general trial court, although in some states the hearing is held before a special quasijudicial agency. At least 16 states at the present time require a jury decision, many of these qualifying this by providing a jury only on request by the patient or someone acting on his behalf. A jury trial is not mandatory in most states. Most of the jurisdictions having judicial commitment recognize that the patient has the right to be represented by counsel at the hearing. However, only about half of the states actually appoint counsel if the patient does not have a lawyer. On the basis of the finding made at the hearing, the patient may be committed for an indeterminate period of time or discharged.

Involuntary hospitalization for an indeterminate period of time can also be accomplished through two other procedures. Most of the time, hospitalization results from *medical certification.* Over 30 jurisdictions in this country allow for hospitalization by this method. Certification can be made by one or most often two physicians, although the decision of these physicians to hospitalize the patient may require the approval of a judge; nonetheless, the procedure is different from judicial hospitalization. In the case of medical certification, the judge is not reviewing whether or not the patient should be admitted but instead is concerned with the genuineness of the documents and the qualifications of the physicians signing the certificates. All of the states permitting medical certification proceedings also permit either the release of the patient on his request after a short period of time or the right of the patient to have his certification reviewed by a court. In most of the states, the patient may be hospitalized against his objections under medical certification for an indeterminate period of time unless he demands a court review. Several states, however, do not allow commitment through medical certification if the patient protests.

The second form of nonjudicial involuntary hospitalization is by an *administrative procedure.* A board consisting for the most part of physicians investigates whether a person is mentally ill and should be hospitalized, and then holds a hearing to determine if he should be committed. Some of the states require a judge or attorney be a member of the administrative board of the hospital, but this is not uniformly the case. Hospitalization through administrative process is often compulsory and can be effected even though the patient objects to the decision.

In addition to the major considerations of who has the authority to commit a patient and what procedures are available for immediate and long-term detention, our hypothetical case raises several significant questions.

1) What degree of illness is required to justify involuntary commitment? It is important to remember that the justification for commitment of a patient is not based simply on a medical decision. In addition to using commitment as a way of treating the patient, the justification for confinement of an individual involves social issues such as the value of removing from the community those who could be dangerous to persons or property. The use of commitment for societal benefit

was a concept well developed in the common law. Following the colonial period, as we discussed in chapter one, states developed statutes to define those circumstances under which an individual could be committed. Of those states now regulating involuntary hospitalization, only a small number limit the criteria for hospitalization to the common law standard of whether a person is potentially dangerous to himself or others in society (See Cross vs Harris, 1969). Several states or jurisdictions have added additional conditions to involuntary commitment. One such condition, found in nearly 20 states, is that commitment is appropriate if predicated on the patient's need for treatment or hospital care. Interestingly, some states have this criterion as the only condition justifying involuntary commitment. And in a few states, for example Colorado, the definition of what constitutes mental illness includes not only persons afflicted with mental disease, but also the infirm and the aged. Also, these statutes permit confinement if it can be shown to be for the "welfare" of either the individual himself or others in society, and their definitions of welfare do not always require that a patient be dangerous to others. But perhaps the broadest definition of what constitutes a condition warranting involuntary commitment is found in the Massachusetts statute (1965) which includes in its definition those who might be classified as nonconformist: "Mentally ill person, for the purpose of involuntary commitment . . . shall mean . . . [one who] is likely to conduct himself in the manner which clearly violates the established laws, ordinances, conventions or morals of the community."

It is apparent, therefore, that dangerousness to self or others, the common law determinant, has been expanded to include "for the welfare of others" and behaviors which, though not dangerous, could be classified as simply not in conformance with the norms of the community. The description therefore of a mentally ill person who qualifies for involuntary commitment is very broad, calling into question the appropriateness of using an instrument for confinement where due process of law can so easily be avoided. It could be strongly argued that where judicial hospitalization is operative and a hearing is required as well as the presence of legal counsel, the Constitutional rights of the individual against unwarranted incarceration are safeguarded. Where in fact medical certification or even administrative commitment are the primary sources for involuntary commitment, then the legality of vague definitions which include even those described simply as nonconformist is questionable. In effect, the degree of mental illness which justifies commitment—and this includes voluntary as well as involuntary commitment—is not clearly defined in any of the statutes save those which limit commitment to persons who are demonstrably potentially harmful to themselves or others.[*]

2) Are others besides the mentally ill susceptible to involuntary commitment? As Kittrie (1971) has pointed out in *The Right to Be Different*, there seems to be a growing trend toward using the treatment model rather than criminal sanctions in dealing with various deviant groups in the population. Provisions exist in over 30 states for the hospitalization of the chronic alcoholic and the drug addict. In fact, in the District of Columbia, as we have already discussed in Chapter 3, the chronic alcoholic is no longer subjected to the criminal process but rather is channeled into a therapeutic program. Similarly, drug addicts, as a result of the Robinson case, are no longer classified as criminals because of their addiction but instead are placed in treatment programs.

One of the difficulties in discussing the alcoholic and the drug addict in this

See Addendum, p. 159.

section is that the degree of alcoholism or even drug addiction which warrants commitment is never clearly defined. The only existing definition describes the chronic alcoholic as one who has reached the point of habitual use of alcohol and has virtually lost the power of self-control in regard to such beverages. Often included in this definition is the additional statement that his alcoholism endangers the welfare of himself or others in society. In some states this definition is not sufficient; instead they require that an individual be convicted of the offense of intoxication at least once before he can be classified as an alcoholic subject to involuntary commitment. In states without separate provisions for involuntary commitment of the alcoholic or drug addict, these individuals may be included under the provision for the commitment of the mentally ill. In fact, some states actually include drug addiction in the definition of mental illness, the reasoning being that drug addicts lose their capacity for self-control.

In addition to chronic alcoholics and drug addicts, involuntary commitment is also justified in many states for epileptics, the mentally deficient, and as already mentioned, the aged and senile. With the advent of drugs that effectively control the seizures of epilepsy, the epileptic is rarely hospitalized through involuntary commitment. The mentally deficient person, classified as such on the basis of some defect in mental development either congenital or evolving during the first few years of life, is still subject to involuntary commitment. Again, the definition of a mentally deficient person in many states includes any person who is incapable of controlling or managing his conduct. As we have seen in the chapter on patient rights, there is an increasing emphasis at the present time on the civil rights, especially the right to receive an education while in an institution, of mentally deficient persons, as they represent a large percentage of those involuntarily committed.

3) Can involuntary commitment ever be avoided if the patient protests? Under certain conditions as defined by the statutes in several states an individual may be committed for hospitalization if he does not register an objection, this type of commitment often being referred to as "nonprotesting" commitment because if the patient protested, he would have to be released immediately. The difference between a nonprotesting admission and the usual involuntary commitment that that in the latter the decision is compulsory on the patient, and despite his protests, he is required to remain in the institution either a determinate period of time or until a judicial review is conducted. On the other hand, the nonprotesting admission can be distinguished from "voluntary" admission in that the patient has not requested admission on his own but is presented for admission by a relative, friend or physician. In several states, involuntary commitment through medical certification is of the nonprotesting variety; that is to say, if the patient objects to the admission, he must be immediately released or shortly thereafter. Nonprotested admissions are considered especially desirable because they avoid both the delay created by a formal hearing on the determination of the mental state of the patient and the exposure of the patient to psychiatrically injurious evaluation.

4) What constitutes voluntary admission? Voluntary admission means those admissions to a mental facility requested by the patient himself, or in the case of a minor or mentally defective, by someone who has been designated by the law to act on the patient's behalf. There has been a significant increase in recent years of voluntary admissions. In the past, involuntary commitment to a mental institu-

tion was the way most patients entered mental hospitals. The trend has definitely shifted toward voluntary admissions; at the present time nearly half of all admissions to mental institutions are initiated by the patient himself. Most states have statutes which regulate very closely admission of the mentally ill to a hospital under voluntary conditions. Merely the desire to enter a hospital does not guarantee the patient's admission. Mental health institutions have broad discretionary powers to either admit or reject patients based on the perception of the physician that the individual will not benefit from treatment or on the limited facilities for handling patients. Some states have instituted a process of informal voluntary admission that doesn't require the patient to submit a formal application in writing. One advantage of voluntary admission over involuntary commitment is that it does give the patient considerable power over determining when he can terminate treatment. This will be discussed in further detail in a later chapter.

5) Considering the legal issues surrounding civil commitment of the mentally ill, are there alternatives which would serve the same medical and social purposes as hospitalization? Probably the most significant advance in recent years in the area of mental health has been the development of effective tranquilizing medication such as thorazine. With the controlled use of such medication, patients are able to live relatively normal lives without having to be hospitalized. Perhaps the biggest impact of tranquilizing medication has been on the behavior of the so-called violent patient, that patient who would meet the common law requirement for commitment. (The Common Law is a combination of English and American laws developing from decisions based on custom and precedent.) In addition to such medication, the concept of the community mental health care system has developed to encourage patients to remain in the home context using the mental health center on an out-patient basis. In some programs hospitals are used only on a daytime basis so patients can return home at night and experience the beneficial influences of living in society.

Many psychiatrists are convinced that involuntary commitment of certain classes of individuals such as the aged, senile, and the so-called "nonconformist," is unjust. Involuntary commitment seriously intrudes upon the rights of the individual and therefore should be limited to extreme circumstances such as when there is a likelihood that the patient may be dangerous to himself or others. Clearly, there is no justification for denying an individual his rights simply because he is old or because he does not conform to societal notions of appropriate behavior. In the case of the chronic alcoholic or drug addict, involuntary commitment is justifiable only when treatment is provided.

Furthermore, and some states already require this, there should be frequent review of patients who have been involuntary committed. Periodic review by medical staff as well as judicial bodies discourages the abuse of the provision for indeterminate detention. In fact it would be more consistent with maintaining the civil rights of citizens to construct a system whereby indeterminate detention is never allowed; medical authorities and the courts should periodically be forced to justify detention.

The present system of involuntary commitment does not sufficiently safeguard the rights of patients. In addition to requiring periodic review of the status of the patient, the definition of the degree of mental illness that qualifies for involuntary commitment should be more clearly circumscribed. Statutes with definitions of mentally ill that include those who are not psychotic or dangerous to others are so vague in their classification they are an infraction of the Constitutional rights of many citizens.

In conclusion, therefore, there should be a very close alignment between the use of involuntary commitment and the ends that are to be served by such hospitalization. Patients who can be treated more effectively outside the hospital should not be committed, and involuntary commitment under any condition should be for determinate periods of time with frequent reviews of the patient's progress.

REFERENCES

Brakel SJ, Rock RS (1971): The Mentally Disabled and the Law (revised ed). Chicago, University of Chicago Press pp. 17–132

Chambers D L (1972): Alternatives to civil commitment of the mentally ill: Practical guide and constitutional imperatives. Michigan Law Rev 70:1107

Colorado Revised Statutes Annotated (1964), 71-1-1-(b)

Cross vs Harris, (1969) 418 F 2d 1095 (In this case the U.S. Court of Appeals for the District of Columbia felt that the mere possibility of "injury to others" was too broad, and required instead that harm be "likely.")

Hutt P, Merrill R (1968–1969): Criminal responsibility and the right to treatment for intoxication and alcoholism. Georgetown Law Rev 57:835

Kittrie N (1971): The Right to Be Different. Baltimore, Johns Hopkins Press

Livermore JM, Malmquist CP, Meehl PE (1968): On the justifications for civil commitment. University of Pennsylvania Law Rev 117:75

Massachusetts Annotated Laws, (1965) 123 Section 1

Note (1967): Civil restraint, mental illness and the right to treatment. Yale Law J 77:87

Projects (1967): Civil commitment of the mentally ill. UCLA Law Rev 14:822

Rock R S (1968): Hospitalization and the Discharge of the Mentally Ill. Chicago, The University of Chicago Press

Ross A (1959): Commitment of the mentally ill: Problems of law and policy. Michigan Law Rev 57:945

Shah SA (1975): Dangerousness and civil commitment of the mentally ill: Some public policy considerations. Am J Psychiat 132:501

6 CONFIDENTIALITY

Safeguarding a patient's right to confidentiality in all matters related to psychiatric treatment, including even the fact that a patient is in therapy or in a hospital is the responsibility of every mental health professional. Not only might revelation of information given in therapy damage a patient's reputation or impede his ability to obtain a job or other position in the community (as was revealed in a recent presidential campaign in the instance of a vice-presidential candidate), but it is also necessary to provide an atmosphere that will permit candor in therapy that assists both therapist and patient to arrive at insights into why the patient continues maladaptive behaviors.

Today confidentiality is becoming all the more important as the psychiatric clinician is increasingly pressed to provide information to various agencies that demand, (and in some cases with good reason) information about a patient's history, diagnosis, treatment and prognosis. While there are clearly outlined procedures which allow the release of varying amounts of information on a patient's written and signed request that free the clinician from legal responsibility, the therapist should still be aware of the multiple ramifications of release of information. All wish to believe that each individual's right to privacy is respected by the professional person; but in this century sophisticated methods of extracting information have been developed (including electronic devices used for wire tapping, recorders to tape conversations without an individual's knowledge, and large computer data banks that carry information gathered at all points during the trajectory of an individual's life.) These, in malevolent hands, threaten an individual's right to privacy. Many more people are involved in processing information in large hospitals and psychiatric clinics than ever before; committees formed to review patient flow, treatment policies, and financing of care involve many people hired to extract information for statistical and billing purposes. Although such data may be used legitimately for studies that ultimately improve care this is another break in the line of privacy. Secretaries, aides, administrators, receptionists and other individuals who do not have a vested interest in safeguarding privacy are yet another threat to a patient's confidentiality.

There are several individuals and agencies who may legitimately request information about some aspect of a patient's psychiatric care of a clinician, with the patient's permission. In most cases a simple guideline is to reveal as little information as possible and to discuss with the patient what that material will be.

If a patient is seeking care from another physician or therapist, obviously the amount of information concerning previous treatment will be greater than if an insurance company desires to legitimize a claim. The same would be true of a hospital seeking a summary of a patient's previous treatment, as this would have direct bearing on the patient's treatment. A requestor may need less personal history or diagnostic information and more prognostic data. Employers may be concerned about an employee's ability to function at a given job or under certain dangerous or risky conditions (*e.g.*, driving a school bus, operating a welding machine, working in a high security agency). An educational institution may need to know if a student will be able to assume the responsibility and stresses of class work, graduate or professional school. Municipal agencies may need employability information to legitimize a request to be placed on the welfare role or a request for a certain type of home care arrangement (e.g., a mother's aid to help with children). Members of a patient's family may desire information about the genetics of a disease and a professional opinion as to whether children will be "tainted." A husband may wonder if his wife will be able to care for her children. A wife may wonder if she will have to become the major source of income for a family. Or any family member of friend may wonder about potentiality for suicide or homicide, or query what they can do to facilitate a patient's functioning and to minimize those sources of stress which aggravate a patient's condition. Finally, a psychiatric clinician may be called upon to testify in court in a variety of capacities which may involve aspects of what has been communicated to him by his patient.

HYPOTHETICAL CASE EXAMPLE: L.C., a 61-year-old white, single, Jewish librarian for a private foundation was informed that the new director, a much younger man, was replacing her with an individual of his own choosing. L.C. had conceptualized the organization of the library for which she had been praised. Unfortunately, L.C. had no independent income and the loss of her job would mean not only a loss of income making it necessary for her to go on welfare, but the loss of retirement benefits to which she would be entitled in four years when she would be 65. The woman felt she was being discriminated against in favor of a younger woman who was a friend of her new director. She contacted a lawyer who found that government grants had been given to the foundation and therefore certain employment practices were required. He requested a Labor Department investigation of the situation and found that the firing of his client was clearly illegitimate. The new director, however, was informed by another employee that L.C. had been under psychiatric care since the death of her mother five months before.

The director stated, therefore, that he had terminated the patient's employment because he felt she was becoming senile. His attorney suggested that L.C.'s psychiatric records be subpoenaed in an attempt to show that she was unstable.

DISCUSSION

This hypothetical case introduces the topic of "privileged communication" as it exists between patients and their physicians. The patient in the case described has the right in many jurisdictions throughout this country to prevent the physician from disclosing information about her without her consent during a court proceeding. This privileged communication between a physician and patient was unknown to Common Law and therefore does not exist unless there is a statute which provides the patient with this right. Over 30 states at the present time have such a statute which, in effect, recognizes that communication made by a patient to his physician in the course of medical treatment is confidential and can not be divulged by the physician during litigation. These statutes, therefore, are concerned with restricting disclosure of confidential information during testimony. They do not deal with the question of whether the physician has an obligation to treat the information imparted to him by his patient as confidential and therefore, not to be transmitted to others not involved with the court proceeding. This question of the physician's obligation to respect the confidentiality of personal information outside court proceeding involves specific Common Law principles and will be discussed later in this chapter.

Physician–patient privilege emerged because society has significantly greater interest in encouraging those who need medical care for either physical or mental conditions freely to obtain it than in soliciting information which may be important for the resolution of a civil or criminal action. In keeping with this then, the physician–patient privilege is structured to preclude the disclosure by a physician of information which has been communicated to him by a patient and which could possibly result in shame or disgrace or other injury to that patient. This privilege, therefore, specifically prohibits the disclosure of that information which has been revealed to the physician in connection with the illness of the patient. In the case of the diabetic patient, such a privilege would forbid the physician from revealing that the patient has diabetes, the period of time he has had the condition, the nature of treatment and prognosis. With regard to psychotherapy where the social and interpersonal history of the patient is a major aspect of the treatment, virtually everything the patient discloses is "privileged" and cannot be revealed under testimony unless the patient explicitly waives his rights of confidentiality. If, however, a physician learns some interesting fact about a patient at a social gathering, it could be argued strongly that such information is not within the physician–patient relationship and, therefore, would not be treated as privileged information.

Congress has not passed a statute establishing the right of privileged communication between the physician and the patient in federal courts. However, the federal rules of evidence for federal courts which are promulgated by the Supreme Court of the United States, include the provision for privileged communication between a patient and a psychotherapist. Federal rules of evidence of course only apply to federal courts, and as we have already discussed, well over 30 states have passed statutes allowing for privileged communication. The California statute for privileged communication is reasonably representative of the statutes which exist in the other states though it would be important to examine carefully the statutes of each jurisdiction for the precise definition of the nature of the privilege varies. This statute also prohibits disclosure of confidential material even outside the court room, unless it is for the benefit of the patient.

> "As used in this article, Confidential Communication Be-
> tween Patient and Physician means information including
> information obtained by an examination of the patient,
> transmitted between a patient and his physician in the
> course of that relationship and in confidence by a means
> which, so far as the patient is aware, discloses the informa-
> tion to no third-person other than in consultation of those
> to whom disclosure is reasonably necessary for the trans-
> mission of the information for the accomplishment of the
> purpose for which the physician is consulted and includes
> the diagnosis made and the advice obtained by the physi-
> cian in the course of that relationship" (California Evi-
> dence Code Annotated, 1972).

This communication rule as framed in nearly all states applies to licensed physicians. Lay analysts who have not obtained a medical degree and are not qualified for licensure, may be compelled on a witness stand to relate intimate information concerning their patients. Similarly, nurses and psychiatric social workers are not obligated to the requirements of privileged communication unless they are acting as agents of the physician in the care of specific patients. Privileged communication, therefore, requires the presence of a physician–patient relationship. If a physician merely examines a patient for a third party or perhaps the court, or observes the patient while he is in confinement, the privilege does not apply because the physician–patient relationship has not been established. The situation changes however if the physician administers treatment to the patient, for this act clearly creates a "contractual" relationship between the physician and the patient. With regard to the relationship between staff physicians and inmates of mental health institutions, the physician–patient relationship does exist and all conditions regarding privileged communication are operative.

Restricting the rule of privileged communication to licensed physicians is not a unanimous stipulation among the states possessing a privileged communication statute. New York Civil Rights Law passed in 1972, gives the broadest possible coverage to those individuals involved in the care of patients. It applies the notion of privileged communication to psychologists, nurses and social workers, when testifying in trials as well as physicians. It is important to note, however, that the confidential information belongs to the patient not the mental health practitioner and if he consents to having information brought out at a court proceeding, the mental health practitioner cannot refuse his request.

The right of the patient to confidentiality of information is not an unrestricted right. Some states disregard the privileged communication rule where there is a strong public policy for the disclosure of information and where it is necessary for the proper administration of justice. There is a variety of situations where it would be appropriate to eliminate the privileged communication rule. If the patient, for example, is suffering from a venereal disease or has been procuring narcotics illegally, disclosure of such information to the appropriate health authorities is essential for the protection of society in general. Similarly, in some cases the privileged communication rule has no effect on the disclosure of psychiatric information as with a parent during a custody hearing, or the driver of an automobile while under the influence of alcohol charged with involuntary manslaughter. Some courts actually achieve the same results by deciding in specific cases that a physician–patient relationship had not been established, and, therefore, the communication would not be protected as privileged by the statute.

Although central to the hypothetical case, the rule of privileged communications is not the only significant feature involving confidentiality of patient information. There are other important issues raised indirectly by this case.

1) Is the patient protected from confidential communication being imparted by his physician to a third party under circumstances other than in a court proceeding?

There have been ethical proscriptions against the disclosure by a physician of his patients' "secrets" since the time of Hippocrates. The Hippocratic Oath specifically prohibits divulging personal information: ". . . whatever, in connection with my professional practice or not in connection with it, I see or hear, in the life of men, which ought not to be spoken abroad, I will not divulge, as reckoning that all such should be kept secret . . ." In the Principles of Medical Ethics promulgated by the American Medical Association, this obligation of the physician to preserve the confidentiality of information learned in the patient–physician relationship has been strongly reinforced. The only exceptions to this rule of secrecy arise in situations where the disclosure of personal information protects the welfare of the individual or society in general. In all other cases, a physician's decision unrestrictively to reveal intimacies about patients is considered a serious infraction against his ethics as a practitioner of medicine.

In addition to his ethical sanctions the physician could also be held liable if he communicated personal information to a third party, particularly in those states in which the physician has a legal obligation not to disclose confidential information and is subject to the charge of libel or slander if he does. Libel is the conveying of information which creates an unjustly unfavorable impression about the patient, and slander is a gross misrepresentation or false assertion and invasion of privacy. Like the ethical sanctions the legal obligations can be circumvented if there is a compelling reason, the protection of the welfare of the individual or of the community. When overriding circumstances prevail, the physician assumes the responsibility of disclosing intimacies about his patient, but he must assure that it is done in good faith with reasonable care, that what is being conveyed is true, that the information is reported fairly and that only the minimum amount of information is communicated and only to the necessary individuals. Of course, if the patient has given prior consent to the physician then there is no legal obligation for the physician to refrain from disclosing the necessary facts.

The following are a few examples of situations which justify the disclosure of confidential information:

    A. Reporting diseases. If the physician knows a patient has a contagious or infectious disease, he is not held liable in damages if he informs those closest to the patient that the patient is so afflicted. There have been several cases where the court held that the physician was justified in informing a variety of individuals a patient had venereal disease. In one case, the physician was considered justified in telling a hotel manager that a patient suffered from a venereal disease; in another no liability was found when an employer was informed of a similar serious communicable disease.

In addition, most states require by statute that the department of health be informed of communicable diseases as well as drug dependency. For example, the Ohio statute requires that physicians and hospitals report contagious disease as soon as possible to the department of health of that state. With regard to drug dependencies, some states, Connecticut for example, require that each practitioner of medicine must report to the commissioner of health the name, address and date of birth of every person who might be dependent upon drugs.

B. Disclosure to spouses. Under most conditions, physicians can disclose the medical condition of a husband or wife to the other spouse without breaking the rule of confidential communication. The courts of several states have maintained that each spouse has the right to know of the presence of a disease that affects the other partner.

There has been at least one case in recent years where the court held that the physician did not commit a breech of confidentiality when at the request of the parents of a prospective bride, he revealed information about the psychiatric history of her fiance causing the parents to withdraw their consent to the marriage. The court felt that the well-being and interests of another were in jeopardy.

C. Reports to agencies, governmental and other institutions. For the most part the courts have felt that a physician does not violate the confidentiality of private communication by submitting a patient's medical records to an agency that has a legitimate interest in this information. Such agencies include schools as well as the patient's employer. Should it be shown, however, that the physician possessed malicious intent in disclosing this information even to legitimate agencies, he could then be held responsible for unethical conduct. Malicious intent might be present if the information disclosed is inaccurate and he refuses on request to retract specific injurious statements.

2) In light of the expanded use of the computer in storing and retrieving information about patients, are there ways of preventing the indiscriminate disclosure of confidential information on medical records?

Concern about computerized data systems has increased considerably in recent years. In an address given before the American Medical Association, President Ford, then vice-president, emphasized the privacy of medical records particularly if Congress would enact some form of national health insurance in the near future. In the area of psychiatric information the need for protecting medical records from indiscriminate disclosure is particularly crucial. Information gathered about psychiatric patients involves the most sensitive issues in a person's private life; therefore, such data must be afforded the strictest confidentiality and be virtually inaccessible except for authorized purposes.

The development of the Multi-State Information System for Psychiatric Patient Records (MSIS), already a collection of records from at least seven states, brings into focus the need for controls of computerized information, over and above the existing Common Law remedies for invasion of privacy, libel or slander. Perhaps one way to achieve maximum control is to require the patient's consent for any information that is to be disclosed by the computer. In the MSIS system passwords are necessary in order to obtain information about any person whose data has been computerized. One of the states involved in this pilot program, New York, passed special legislation in 1972 placing significant impediments in the way of obtaining the psychiatric records in the computerized MSIS system. This act prevents courts and other administrative bodies from obtaining these records even with a subpoena. Most of the states not involved in the MSIS system are still in the very early stages of developing data processing methods for more efficient retrieval of patient data.

Many states have passed legislation which assures the confidentiality of psychiatric records in mental health facilities, except for purposes of psychiatric research and epidemiological studies. In these cases in many states there can be no disclosure of information which might identify the patient, and data are restricted to authorized personnel. With the emergence of more multistate, computerized systems, significantly more efficient than the existing methods for information storage and retrieval, many states are likely to follow the example set by New York and pass statutes to control more closely disclosure of computerized data.

3) What is the underlying theory for the requirement that medical information be confidential?

The relationship of the psychiatric clinician to the patient is one of trust; the patient places himself in the care of the psychiatric clinician with the expectation that the physician will not only give him a high quality care but will also be loyal and maintain his privacy. He gives the psychiatric clinician considerable power and control over him by revealing the most vulnerable aspects of his personal life. But this power is not without its reservations for also stipulated is the responsibility to safeguard his interests and under certain conditions prefer that interest unless there is the possibility of harm to the patient or society. The physician–patient relationship, therefore, is an intimate relationship, an arrangement that is so important that the law recognizes the seriousness of the physician's responsibilities. His obligations to the patient are comparable in some respects to the responsibilities that an officer of a large corporation has to the interests of the corporation and specifically the stockholders. This relationship in a corporation is referred to as a *fiduciary* or trust relationship. Similarly, society invests psychiatric clinicians with the responsibilities of a fiduciary relationship to their patients. The status of the relationship between a clinician and a patient, therefore, demands trust, loyalty and the confidentiality of information essential for the patient's interest.

4) Does a patient have the right to his own psychiatric records? Psychiatrists for the most part retain the right to decide if they should release medical information to a patient. The psychiatrist's records contain more than just factual information about a patient. They often include the patient's perceptions about his environment and the psychiatrist's evaluations, both of which are highly subjective and could have a detrimental affect on the patient who hears these things. The decision to release records must therefore take into account the affect that such information might have on the patient, as well as its potential benefit to the patient or society. If the patient consents, directors of public and private institutions usually release that information which is specifically at issue in a trial or administrative procedure. Rarely is the complete record released unless subpoenaed by a court.

If the psychiatrist refuses to release psychiatric information about a patient, the patient can bring the issue to court. If the matter is of importance in a trial, the court will likely require that the information be released. In a recent court case in California the defendant asked his psychiatrist to disclose information about his mental and emotional condition. The psychiatrist refused despite the request of the court and was held in contempt, risking a possible jail sentence (In re Lifschutz, 1972). The California Supreme Court held in this case that there was no need for absolute confidentiality in the psychotherapist–patient relationship and gave the judge the power to decide what information would be important to assure a just verdict.*

REFERENCES

Berry vs March, (1958) 8 Utah 2d 191, 331 P 2d 814

California Evidence Code Annotated (1972), Section 992 West Supp—as amended Stat (1972), C 650 p 2006 Section 4

Castiglioni A (1947): A History of medicine. New York, Alfred A. Knopf

Cochran vs Sears-Roebuck, (1945) 34 SE 2d 296, (GA)

Connecticut General Statutes Annotated (1958), Title 19: 333, Public Health & Safety, Section 19–48a

Connecticut General Statutes 52–146d–146f

Curran WJ, Laska EM, Kaplan H, Bank R (1973): Protection of privacy and confidentiality. Science 182: 797

Dawidoff D (1973): The Malpractice of Psychiatrists. Illinois, Charles C. Thomas

Dawidoff D (1966): The malpractice of psychiatrists, Duke Law J 1966:696

Disclosure of confidential information, (1971). *JAMA* 216:385

Entralgo P L (1969): Doctor and Patient. New York, McGraw Hill

Gustafson vs Gustafson, (1968) 158 SE 2d 619, NC

Guttmacher, M, Weihofen H (1952): Psychiatry and the Law. New York, WW Norton

In re Lifschutz, (1970) 2 Calif 3d 330

Keeping the patient's secrets (1966). *JAMA* 195:227

Kline NS, Laska E (ed) (1968): Computer & Electronic Devices in Psychiatry. New York, Grune & Stratton

Legal aspects of computerized medical records, (1968). *JAMA* 205:153

McGarry, Al, Kaplan, HA (1973): Overview: Current trends in mental health law. Am J Psychiatry 130:621–630

Morse HN (1971): The tort liability of the psychiatrist, Baylor Law Rev. 19:208

New York Civil Rights Law, (1972) Act 45, Sections 4501, 4507, 4508

News Note Address by Vice President Ford to AMA (June 26, 1974) Washington Post, p. A–2

Ohio Revised Code Annotated, (1964) Section 3701.24 (Baldwin)

Plaut, EA (1974): A perspective on confidentiality. Am J Psychiatry 131: 1021–1024

Privileged communications statutes (1969). JAMA 207:1415

Privileged communications statutes (1968). JAMA 197:257

Simonsen vs Swenson, (1920) 177 NW 831 (NB)

State of North Carolina vs Hollingsworth, (1964) 139 SE 2d 235

State of North Carolina vs Howard, (1968) 158 SE 2d 350, NC

*See Addendum, p. 159.

THE PATIENT'S RIGHTS
7 WHILE
IN THE HOSPITAL

A common misconception of the lay public is that admission to a mental hospital entails abdication of one's civil rights. The loss of such rights as the right to make a contract, the right to marry and divorce and the right to buy and dispose of property are fortunately not easily lost. There are situations, however, that release a psychiatric patient from certain obligations while he is acutely psychotic, or in other instances he may be forbidden to perform certain legal functions because of a psychiatric disturbance, be it a psychogenic or organic psychosis or mental subnormality. Obviously an important consideration is the mental status of a patient at the time he attempts to, or if the transaction has already been performed, when he attempted to exercise a legal right. Friends and relatives may in retrospect have varying opinions as to the patient's mental status; a patient himself may on recovery realize that he committed an act of poor judgment, or, regretting an action performed when his judgment was actually intact attempt to clear himself of any responsibility. This may be the reasoning of a psychiatric outpatient with a relatively mild problem. He wishes to recover a financial loss from a bad investment made when he was depressed but not sufficiently so to be considered so severely mentally unstable not to be held legally responsible for his financial obligations. Comparably, a person may wish to annul a marriage contracted under similar circumstances. When the patient is in a hospital his right to exercise certain rights may relate to the type of hospitalization (*viz.* voluntary or involuntary), in addition to his mental status.

HYPOTHETICAL CASE EXAMPLE: P.R., a 32-year-old white, separated, Protestant businessman, was admitted voluntarily to a private psychiatric hospital following five days of grandiose and manic behavior. The patient had a family history of three generations of manic–depressive illness, and he himself had an episode of mania at age 23, one month before he was to complete work on a Masters of Business Administration, and an episode of depression at age 28 without any discernible precipitant. Following the second episode, he was placed on lithium carbonate and was free of any recurrence for four years. Five months prior to admission, he moved from a large southern city where he was in an administrative role in a branch of a large firm to take a comparable position in the company's main office in New York. He had requested the transfer when he and his wife of eight years decided to obtain a legal separation. He had been told by his former psychiatrist in the South to contact the psychiatrist in New York City with whom his therapist had trained. As he was busy getting an apartment in New York and with new responsibilities in his home office, he neglected to make contact and ran out of medication. Two months later and five days prior to admission, he began to propose massive plans for reform in his company's policy and suggested that he personally assume the role of director so that a bountiful future for the company be assured. On the day of admission he had summoned a meeting of the board of directors to outline his "new plan." The corporation's president, aware both of the patient's tremendous capacity to perform solid work when not ill and of his past psychiatric history, convinced the patient to see a psychiatrist and admit himself to a hospital if necessary. He was guaranteed his job would be waiting for him when he was discharged.

After being in the hospital two weeks, the patient decided to continue a transaction with a local real estate agent he had begun several weeks prior to hospitalization. He had inherited considerable acreage in Vermont which he wished to sell before he obtained a divorce from his wife. He summoned the realtor, who arrived on the hospital ward with a lawyer. He was convinced by the realtor and the lawyer, a good friend of the realtor, that the land was not so valuable as the patient originally thought, and the patient agreed to sell it at a price considerably less than that originally quoted to him by other realtors. Two months after discharge, he regretted the sale and decided to contest the contract because he signed it while in a mental hospital. Is the sale valid?

DISCUSSION

The important issue in this case is concerned with how "incompetency" is established, particularly the effect that hospitalization has in that determination. Incompetency usually refers to situations where an individual has been judged incapable of making knowledgeable transactions or of managing his own property and business affairs. The patient in this hypothetical illustration, voluntarily admitted to the mental hospital, was not designated to be incompetent through a judicial proceeding. The question of whether hospitalization *per se* suggests incompetency is a complicated one. In the case of the voluntarily admitted patient, as in the example, there would appear to be no relationship between hospitalization and incompetency. In fact not only are there no state statutes which create such a relationship, but also a few states, Texas in particular, contain statutory provisions that specifically state that voluntary patients are to lose none of their civil rights during the course of hospitalization.

This is not to say, however, that voluntary patients are not denied their civil rights, such as the right to contract. Several states have statutes which allow mental institutions the power to restrict the legal functions of patients. These statutes exist despite the fact that there are no provisions directly relating voluntary admission to incompetency. An example of such a provision is in the Utah Code which clearly states that "limitations may be imposed by the hospital" on the legal capacities of the patient. Furthermore, there is no distinction between voluntarily and involuntarily admitted patients from the standpoint of who is susceptible to administrative regulations. These regulations may be established by individual hospitals or by a state-wide system regulating mental health facilities and programs, such as a state department of mental health. And, these regulations possess the added feature of denying the patient recourse for questioning his presumed incompetency to handle his own affairs. In circumstances where a statute has been enacted to deny the incompetent his right to enter into contractual arrangements, the patient could argue before a proper legal forum that he is not "incompetent" and hence should not be denied these important civil rights. On the basis of evidence provided by the patient, the judge might concur with the patient and restore these functions. With regard to administratively imposed regulations the patient is left with no effective recourse to question their decision.

In states where the prerogative is not granted the mental institution, the voluntarily or temporarily admitted patient may not be denied certain legal rights, though confinement may still imply incompetency and administrative regulations may still be operative. The situation is different, however, for the involuntarily committed patient; some states still maintain that an order for indeterminate hospitalization is equivalent to being judged incompetent. Of course, the consensus is against merging the concepts of involuntary commitment with incompetency, and most states have abandoned this principle, though, a few states maintain this relationship. For example, the Ohio statute includes among the various conditions that justify labeling as incompetent those involuntary committed— "incompetent means any person . . . indeterminately hospitalized . . ." The contemporary view of incompetency sees no necessary correlation between a patient needing care and his ability to conduct his personal affairs. According to most state statutes, involuntary admissions are initiated for the purposes of protecting the patient from his own destruction (suicide), protecting others from a patient's lack of control (homicide). and administering needed treatment. The establishment of incompetency is predicated on society's desire to safeguard a patient's assets from his own inability to comprehend the significance of business transactions. The reasons for involuntary commitment and for judging competency are therefore essentially different. Despite the fact that most states separate these concepts into distinct proceedings, the involuntary commitment of a patient in many states still signifies a strong presumption of incompetency and the policies and procedures of hospitals may effectively impose the legal status of "incompetent."

The determination of legal incompetency in states that do not merge incompetency with the need for hospitalization may be done through an independent proceeding, though it may be one of the major issues decided at a commitment proceeding. By the same token, an individual may be considered legally incompetent without being hospitalized since the criteria for involuntary commitment and those for incompetency differ. Persons who may be designated incompetent because they are unable to handle their property and affairs include the mentally ill and mentally deficient in all states, and in some states drug addicts, alcoholics, the elderly and senile. A number of states also include in their statutes a catch-all category of those others who do not fit the descriptions above, but who are unable to manage their property. In most states when an individual is legally described as incompetent, a guardian is usually appointed by a court to oversee his estate.

The guardian is empowered to manage the estate, that is to buy and sell property, engage in contractual agreements for the incompetent and even represent him in legal proceedings. Since the guardian is appointed by a court, he is answerable for his decisions regarding the use of the incompetent's property. Under certain conditions he must actually obtain prior approval from the court, particularly when considering a sale of real property on behalf of the incompetent.

In many states the authority of the guardian goes far beyond management of property giving him the power to initiate involuntary commitment proceedings if the incompetent has not been hospitalized. When the incompetent regains the capacity to manage his own affairs he may be restored to legal competency and can dismiss the guardian either through separate judicial proceeding to establish competency or in some jurisdictions simply by being discharged from a mental hospital. Some of the states allowing restoration through discharge may require the patient to improve, in which case a conditional discharge would not necessarily result in the restoration of competency.

When a patient judged incompetent makes a contract, the issue of its validity, according to most court decisions, rests in part on whether the agreement was made before or after he was classified as incompetent. If a patient judged incompetent enters an agreement, any legal transaction he undertakes is usually considered void. In the event a patient judged incompetent is not provided with a guardian, his contracts would be considered by many courts to be voidable, or the contract may be voided if not beneficial to the incompetent person and if he expressly desires that it be voided. Similarly, many jurisdictions take the position regarding contracts made before the individual is judged incompetent that such agreements are voidable if the court bases its final decision on the circumstances of the arrangements and the individual's wish that they be nullified.

Returning to the hypothetical case, the patient was voluntarily admitted to the mental hospital and was at no time judged "incompetent." Furthermore, administrative regulations did not interfere with his participation in business transactions. The fact that he was hospitalized at the time of the contract would be admitted as evidence of his incompetency in a trial contesting the validity of the agreement, but the courts seem to place little importance on this information; his contract would probably be considered valid in most jurisdictions.

There is much confusion in this whole area. The move away from merging involuntary commitment with incompetence is a good one and should be encouraged in those few remaining jurisdictions that maintain this association. The role of administrative regulations in states that provide for this by statute and those that don't should be carefully examined with a view toward ending this practice except under extreme circumstances when the welfare of the patient is clearly in question. Even under these conditions some mechanism should be employed so that the patient can have some recourse against arbitrary administrative decisions. In this issue it would be far more equitable to examine each patient individually. Rather than a blanket deprivation of a patient's rights, the courts should suspend only those which should be denied for his own benefit.

Although the main issue in this hypothetical case involves the determination of incompetency, it is not the only important consideration regarding the patient's rights while in the hospital.

1) Are there other civil rights that are denied to both hospitalized and nonhospitalized mental patients? Various civil rights besides the right to manage one's own business affairs are affected by mental illness and hospitalization. There are strong

prohibitions against marriage of mentally disabled persons. These prohibitions, found in English common law have become incorporated into the statutes of most states. One reason for this prohibition is that the mentally ill person cannot understand the nature of the marriage contract and therefore is unable to consent truly to this relationship. But, perhaps a more pressing reason from the standpoint of societal benefit rests on the notion that mental illness, whether genetically or environmentally induced, often runs in families. Some states have as their primary rationale for forbidding such marriages the preclusion of children who might be inclined to inherit mental illness.

The main difficulty with statutes prohibiting marriages among the mentally ill is that they are nearly impossible to enforce. In some states violating one of these statutes can result in criminal punishment, not only for the parties immediately involved, but for others who might have directly or indirectly assisted the couple. Such sanctions, however, have not proved to be very effectinve. But the situation is different for the hospitalized patient. Statutes prohibiting marriage of a mentally ill person also include those who are hospitalized for mental illness; these prohibitions can be strictly enforced. Even in the absence of a statute, the hospitalized patient is prevented from getting married by administrative or hospital regulations. To complement the effect of these statutes, most states facilitate divorce for the mentally disabled. This topic will be discussed in a later chapter.

In addition to marriage rights, the mentally disabled may be prevented from voting, driving a car or practicing a profession. The laws do not clearly state—as in statutes prohibiting contracts and marriage—whether the legally incompetent are not allowed to vote or if this prohibition includes those who are hospitalized for mental illness though still legally competent. Even in states that explicitly single out the legally incompetent, the hospitalized patient who is "competent" will probably not be able to vote because of hospital policy. Concerning the right to operate a motor vehicle, the state statutes are again difficult to interpret. Most states will not issue a driver's license to a mentally ill or deficient person; in some states this includes drug addicts and alcoholics. Several states suspend a person's license when he enters a mental institution, whether on a voluntary or involuntary basis, while others require that the patient be involuntarily hospitalized or even judged incompetent before he is denied this right. Again the hospitalized patient is prevented from driving whether there is a statute or not.

A mentally ill patient will probably be prevented from practicing a profession. In the case of the patient who is not hospitalized the professional licensure board has the power to suspend and revoke his license. The hospitalized person will be unable to practice a profession, such as law or medicine, simply because he is physically confined to an institution, in addition to the fact that his license can be revoked. The state laws governing a hospitalized patient vary widely; some states permanently revoke the licenses of both voluntarily and involuntarily admitted patients though others reinstate the privilege once the patient is discharged.

Interestingly, mentally ill persons can sue and be sued in most jurisdictions, the exception being the patient who has been judged incompetent and has been appointed a guardian. The guardian is then often given the right to sue and be sued on behalf of the incompetent person.

2) What important civil rights are denied to the hospitalized patient and to what extent? The hospitalized patient, by virtue of his confinement, is particularly vulnerable. Historically, he has been denied the right to communicate to varying degrees with others outside the institution. To some extent this constraint was

reasonable because mental patients often fabricate happenings in the hospital that might be fearful and offensive to friends and close relatives. However, recognition of the importance of protecting the patient against arbitrary and possibly inappropriate hospital decisions resulted in the enactment of statutes in nearly all the states to permit some patient communication. In some states the right is limited to correspondence with public officials or mental health administrators; in other more enlightened states, such as New York, the patient has the right to unrestricted communication with attorneys. In New York this is achieved through a mental health information service, consisting of an attorney located in the mental hospital for the purpose of providing patients with direct contact for advice and legal assistance. In addition to correspondence many states also permit visitation by family and friends, but hospitals are given considerable discretion over controlling the frequency and duration of such visits.

Perhaps the most highly charged current issue regarding the rights often denied the mentally ill is the right to refuse certain kinds of treatment such as electroshock and psychosurgery, some of which border on the experimental. Not many states have dealt with the subject of electroshock, but a few, such as Michigan and New York, have regulations which require consent from a patient or legally responsible person before electroshock can be administered. Only one or two states, California in particular, actually allow the patient the right to refuse electroshock. Psychosurgery has also been essentially ignored by most of the states. A small number require the consent of the patient, a responsible family member or guardian, except perhaps in emergency situations. Others simply state that notice must be given to the patient or guardian that surgery is planned. But mental hospitals are given much discretion to perform psychosurgery, whereas regulations are stricter with general hospitals where consent is mandatory. Presently, various groups are making an effort to regulate the use of psychosurgery on the mentally ill, especially experimental surgery. The Department of Health, Education and Welfare has recently come forward with regulations for human experimentation proposing, among other things, the establishment of "consent committees" to act as ombudsmen, or patient advocates to protect the rights of vulnerable groups such as the mentally ill and deficient, children and prisoners. The concept of a "consent committee" should possibly be expanded to include the protection of vulnerable groups from a range of treatments that are potentially dangerous, of questionable medical value, and seldom fully understood by patients or their families.

REFERENCES

Allen RC, Ferster FZ, Weinhofen H (1968): Mental Impairment and Legal Incompetency. New Jersey, Prentice Hall

Brakel SJ, Rock RS (1971): The Mentally Disabled and the Law (revised ed). Chicago, University of Chicago Press

Comment (1956): The mentally ill and the law of contracts. Temple Law Rev 29:380

Curran WJ, Shapiro ED (1970): Law, Medicine and Forensic Science. Boston, Little Brown

Davidson HA (1952): Forensic Psychiatry. New York, Ronald Press

Green MD (1940): Public policies underlying the law of mental incompetency. Michigan Law Rev 38:1189

Guttmacher MS, Weihofen H (1952): Psychiatry and The Law. New York, WW Norton

Harper FV (1952): Problems of The Family. Indianapolis, Bobbs-Merrill

Lindman M (ed) (1961): The Mentally Disabled and The Law. Chicago, University of Chicago Press

Mayer EJ (1969): Lawyers in a mental hospital. Ment Hyg 53:14–16

McCoid AH (1957): A reappraisal of liability for unauthorized medical treatment. Minnesota Law Rev 41:381 (Mr)

Note (1956): Real property—validity of conveyance by mental incompetents. Wayne Law Rev 3:73

Note (1970): Restructuring informed consent: Legal therapy for the doctor–patient relationship. Yale Law J 79:1533

New York Mental Hygiene Law, (1964) Section 88 (McKiney Supp)

Ohio Revised Code, (1964) 2111.01 CD (Baldwin)

Ohio Revised Code Annotated, (1964) Section 5123.03 (Baldwin)

Oklahoma Statute Revised Annotated, (1951), tit, 43A section 96

Plante ML (1968): An analysis of "informed consent." Fordham Law Rev 36:639

Protection of Human Subjects (1947). Federal Register 39:18914

Rock RS (1968): Hospitalization and Discharge of The Mentally Ill. Chicago, University of Chicago Press

State vs Solfo, (1960) 58 NJ Super 472, 156 A2d 714

Texas Revised Civil Statute Annotated (1958) 5547–4(a to 1) (Supp 1969)

Utah Code Annotated 64–7–48

8 TESTAMENTARY CAPACITY

A patient's testamentary capacity is his ability to make out a valid will. Psychiatric inpatients are obviously not the only individuals who might ask for a psychiatrist's professional opinion about the legal ability required to write a will. In some circumstances a psychiatrist may be called upon to testify about a person long dead, whom he himself never knew. In such instances he would be presented with a series of hypothetical questions based on evidence about the deceased individual. In more usual circumstances, however, he will be called upon to examine a living individual who intends to make out a will.

HYPOTHETICAL CASE EXAMPLE: A 67-year-old widowed, white, Irish-Catholic father of three and retired fire chief, while an inpatient in a psychiatric hospital for a psychotic depressive episode, decided to draw up a will with his lawyer. At the time of actually writing the will he had recovered from his psychosis although still a patient in the hospital. In the will, he split the bulk of his estate, valued at about $65,000, between his two daughters. A third child, a ne'er-do-well son who quit high school at age 16 to work as a sailor on a merchant ship to South America, was left one dollar. It was well known in the patient's family and in his community that he and his son did not get along. Shortly after leaving the hospital, the patient died of a heart attack. When the will was read, the sailor–son decided to contest it stating that his father wrote it while in a mental hospital. The son's lawyer discovered that the father had been admitted to the hospital under a medical commitment because, in his psychotic depression, he threatened to kill himself by jumping off a local bridge and had refused to voluntarily admit himself to a psychiatric hospital. He was committed, therefore, on the grounds that he was a danger to himself. Is the will valid?

DISCUSSION

The right to dispose of property according to the owner's desires remains one of the most guarded prerogatives in our culture. As a consequence it is very difficult to void a person's will or testament unless that person lacks the power to execute a will, a power given by state statutes, lacks the capacity to make a testament or is under undue and possibly coercive influence. The power to execute a will varies from state to state and is determined by statutes clearly defining the conditions by which a will becomes a legally valid document. The question of undue influence arises if it can be shown that the will actually represents the desires of another person rather than those of the testator. For example, it might be shown that an elderly woman living with the oldest of three children was strongly influenced by that child to leave little or nothing to the other children.

The determination of testamentary capacity or the ability to make a will is of particular interest to the psychiatrist. Does insanity alone prevent the making of a valid will? If not what effect does mental illness have? Throughout history law dealt with this important issue in a variety of ways. In England during the second half of the nineteenth century the attitude toward mental illness and testamentary capacity found a will invalid if there was any degree of mental illness in the patient making the will. In contrast, the law in the United States during that same period upheld wills written by persons with very low mental capacity, *i.e.*, the possession of that amount of understanding sufficient to justify testamentary capacity, notwithstanding that the person might have a mental illness.

The modern view of testamentary capacity emerged from a court decision in the 1870s in England and has been adopted in one form or another by nearly every state. The basic notion behind the contemporary test for testamentary capacity is that it does not preclude a valid will on the basis of mental illness or even mental retardation under certain circumstances. The statutes do require the presence of a "sound mind" but the courts have for the most part interpreted this phrase broadly and have consequently developed a comparatively nonrestrictive test for "soundness." The courts in the various states agree that mental competence for making a will exists if the testator meets the following criteria:

1. He knows the nature of the act he is about to perform.
2. He knows his relationship to those persons who are natural objects of his estate —the names and identity of such persons as well as his relationship to them.
3. He knows the nature and extent of the property which he is about to dispose of.

These three elements in one way or another are considered essential to a valid will. To explain further, knowledge of the act he is performing means he knows that he is signing his will. If a testator was intoxicated or mentally confused and disoriented at the time he signed his will, or perhaps if he died very shortly thereafter, a physician might conclude that he did not know what he was doing and the will would be invalid. In regard to the second element, the testator must know the nature and extent of his property. This does not mean that he needs to know exact details as to the precise amount of land he owns or the current balance in his savings account, but by the same token he cannot have attempted to give away more than he possessed. A patient who wills one million dollars worth of securities when he owns only half as much would be considered incompetent to make a will. And, finally the testator must know his relatives, who they are, their relationship to him, and the claims both legal and moral they may have on his estate, although this does not mean he is obligated to leave parts of his estate to specific relatives. If a testator gives over half of his estate to a spouse who has been dead for several years, then it would be reasonable to assume since the dead have no claim on one's property that the testator does not meet the requirement of "soundness" and, therefore, the will will be invalid.

Just as these three features are essential to a valid will, other considerations such as a prior adjudication of incompetency or even involuntary hospitalization do not necessarily prevent a will from being legally constituted. The determination of incompetence after a will has been executed will not in itself negate the will. At the same time that information can be admitted in a court proceeding as evidence against the validity of the will. The deciding factor would then be the nature and seriousness of the mental condition that resulted in "incompetency"—particularly as related to the ability to execute a will—and the length of time between the signing of the will and the court decision on incompetency. If it can be shown that the patient's mental condition had been substantially unchanged then the adjudication of incompetency might be sufficient to negate the will. However, there have been cases where wills have been upheld despite evidence that the patient was mentally compromised and had been even before the will was executed. Involuntary commitment to a mental institution has even less of an impact on invalidating a will than the establishment of mental incapacity. As with the issue of incompetency, evidence of commitment can be considered at a trial disputing a will, but its impact will be marginal as most courts will lean strongly in the direction of validating the will.

An examination of the relationship between the various forms of mental disease and the legality of wills would probably show no necessary association. The condition, instead, must be such that the testator does not possess the degree of "soundness" to meet the legal criteria for testamentary competency. Therefore, there must be a demonstrable relationship between specific mental dysfunction and the ability of the testator to achieve the legally required conditions of a valid will. Feeblemindedness in itself does not invalidate a will. It would, however, if it could be established, for example, that the testator did not know the nature of the act he was performing, in which case the feeblemindedness would be interfering directly with those events that lead up to the formation of a will.

Similarly, diseases of old age—comprising afflictions that affect the largest class of persons involved with testamentary decisions and disputes—do not by themselves preclude the viability of a will. Wills are often upheld even though they are products of very elderly patients. The qualifications of course would be patients suffering from senile brain disease or severe cerebral arteriosclerosis when there would be obvious impairment of such mental functions as memory, orientation and judgment. For example, a severely senile patient may elect to will his entire fortune to an animal despite the fact that four children and many grandchildren have some claim on his property. Clearly in such a case the presence of dementia, significantly impairing judgment, would weigh heavily against accepting the document as representing the desires of the individual involved.

Alcoholism and drug addiction can also invalidate a will if the conditions impair the ability of the testator to meet the criteria of testamentary capacity; but this is not easy to establish in any given case. An individual may be under the influence of alcohol for most of his life, but if on the day he makes and signs his will he is only mildly or not under the influence of alcohol, then he would most likely be meeting the criteria for testamentary capacity. It would probably be easier to invalidate the will of a chronic alcoholic or drug addict if it can be shown that permanent brain damage has occurred directly affecting testamentary capacity. This would also hold true for systemic diseases such as a malignancy or cerebral vascular disease if these conditions directly affect the individual's ability to meet the legal criteria for a will.

The most interesting mental condition creating debate concerning testamentary capacity exists when the testator suffers from delusions. First of all, the mere presence of a delusion or false belief is of no major significance unless it could conceivably alter the outcome of a will. A well circumscribed delusion that certain racial groups are actively colluding to overthrow the government would likely have little impact on the disposition of an individual's property, unless, of course, someone from that group of suspicious persons is a member of the family. Given that such is unlikely to be the case, it would be fairly safe to assume that the delusion is irrelevant to the disposition of property. The issue becomes muddied however, when one examines beliefs that influence the way a testator might perceive family members. The distinction between a delusion and a false belief that may not be in the realm of a delusion is very imprecise. The fact that a person holds beliefs not shared by others does not in and of itself mean that he suffers from delusions. His assessment of his wife's infidelity, for example, may be incorrect, but that is not to say he is mentally ill. The courts have taken the position that a delusion, or belief that is the product of a disordered mind, exists if that belief has virtually no foundation or evidence in reality and, therefore, is so divergent from common views that no "reasonable" man could hold such a position. Some courts have gone so far to condition that though a belief might be irrational and bizarre, it is not a delusion if it is the result of any facts which can be demonstrated to exist. This last qualification conflicts with psychiatric knowledge which suggests delusions can exist even if they are based on factual information. A paranoid individual might be able to support the statement that when he walks down the street some people stare at him; but, to leap from that observation to the conclusion that these people are part of a conspiracy to deprive him of his property rights would be outside the realm of reasonable explanation. To the psychiatrist the distinction between a delusion and a belief that may be false but not the product of a disordered mind rests to a large extent on the appropriateness of the interpretation of facts.

Delusions are of particular significance if they can be shown to affect the testamentary capacity of the person making a will. An individual who feels that he is being directed to sign a will by some external force would be seen as acting out of coercion and the will would be invalidated. Similarly, delusions of grandeur or poverty affecting the testator's knowledge of the nature and extent of his property or paranoid delusions when he constructs a plot of relatives trying to kill him can support a claim that he lacks testamentary capacity to make a valid will. On the other hand, eccentricity will not negate a will. An individual can believe in extrasensory perception, witchcraft or even be a religious fanatic leaving his fortune to a religious cause and his will would not be invalidated for these reasons alone. Ultimately the important issue to the court is whether the false belief, or delusion, causes the testator to dispose of his property in a different way than he would have otherwise. Strange religious views may reasonably be a feature of a person's belief system, but responding to the demands of spiritual voices would not be part of the testator's normal state and probably would not result in a disposition of personal belongings compatible with his usual desires.

Interestingly, there does exist in the laws of most states a recognition of the possibility of "lucid intervals" in the life of patients who are otherwise so compromised mentally that they lack testamentary capacity. If a will is made during a "lucid interval" when the patient is relatively free of the effects of his mental condition it would probably be considered valid even though the testator might shortly relapse into his illness. To establish that a "lucid interval" did in fact occur it would be prudent to have an otherwise mentally deranged person examined by a psychiatrist during the lucid period when the will is being made.

Returning to the hypothetical case, the argument for invalidating the will would probably be insubstantial. The testator in this case met the criteria for testamentary capacity. He was apparently recovered from his psychotic episode at the time of the writing of the will. In addition he demonstrated a knowledge of the nature and extent of his property, and who were related to him and consequently had some claim on his possessions. The fact that he left his son only one dollar does not invalidate the will; giving one dollar confirmed that he was aware his son was related to him but chose to limit the son's claim in the will. Furthermore the widespread knowledge of his bad relationship with his son further supports the fact that the testator was acting as he would if he were not hospitalized. Two other issues would probably be evaluated in a court dispute, but both would have little weight in negating the will. First, the testator died shortly after making the will. A physician may conclude when a testator dies shortly after signing a will that he may have been disoriented near the end of his life. This interpretation would be valid if the testator suffered from a prolonged illness which resulted in his death. In this case the death from a heart attack had miminal or no relationship to his condition at the time the will was signed. And, second, the testator had been involuntarily committed to the mental hospital. We have already discussed that involuntary commitment *per se* has little effect on the validity of wills; the important consideration is whether the testator meets the three broad criteria for testamentary capacity. Since the testator in this hypothetical case seems to meet those criteria, the will would most likely be valid.

Two other brief questions in addition to the major one regarding testamentary capacity are also raised by the hypothetical case and are of some interest.

1) Is there a difference in the criteria for determining when a will is valid and when a contract is valid? The standards for making a valid contract are more stringent than those for executing a will. Court cases have varied on this issue. Some have held that it takes greater mental acuity to negotiate a contract than it does to make a will; others insist that the two acts are comparable. But the majority see the nature of the two acts as so different that the criteria for deciding their validity must logically be different. The definition of competency or the ability to manage one's own property and business affairs seems to require more mental ability than does meeting the three criteria for making a valid will. In fact an individual can be judged "incompetent" and therefore unable to enter into a contractual relationship, yet still able to make a valid will. To some extent this difference might hinge on the overwhelming importance society places on the right of an individual to dispose of his property as he sees fit. The legal system makes it quite difficult to invalidate a will.

2) When a will is contested is it the obligation of the testator or of the person disputing the will to show that the will does or does not meet the legal criteria for testamentary capacity? In the past the individual claiming that the will was valid had the "burden" of substantiating this claim. Recently in many states the trend

increasingly has been to place the burden on the person contesting the will to prove that it is invalid. It is therefore very difficult to invalidate a will, even when there might be strong evidence that the testator was mentally ill to the point of not meeting the criteria for testamentary capacity or that he was under coercion or undue influence from another. Clearly the policy in the past and presently growing in strength has been to protect, as much as possible, the "sanctity" of wills, *i.e.*, the individual's right to dispose of his property as he wishes.

REFERENCES

Allen RC, Ferster FZ, Weihofen H (1968): Mental Impairment and Legal Incompetency. New Jersey, Prentice Hall

1 Bowe-Parker: Page on Wills, Section 12.42; Barnett, AG (1963): Effect of guardianship of adults on testamentary capacity. 89 ALR 2d 1120

Brakel SJ, Rock RS (1971): The Mentally Disabled and the Law (revised ed.). Chicago, University of Chicago Press

Curran WJ, Shapiro ED (1964): Law Med Forensic Sci. Boston, Little Brown

Davidson HA (1965): Forensic Psychiatry. New York, Ronald Press

Epstein J (1962): Testamentary capacity, reasonableness and family maintenance: a proposal for meaningful reform. Temple Law Q 35: 231

Estate of Wolf, (1959) 174 Cal A 2d 144, 344 P 2d 37

Fuller LL, Braucher R (1964): Basic Contract Law. St Paul, West Publishing

In re Knight's Will, (1959) 250 NC 634, 109 SE 2d 470

In re Sommerville, (1962) 406 Pa 207, 177 A 2d 496

In re White's will, (1957) 2 NY 2d 309, 141 NE 2d 416

Overholser W (1959): Major principles of forensic psychiatry, American Handbook of Psychiatry. Edited by S Arieti. New York, Basic Books

Note (1953): Psychiatric assistance in the determination of testamentary capacity. Harvard Law Rev 66:1116

Siegal L (1963): Forensic Medicine. New York, Grune & Stratton

Usdin GL (1957): The physician and testamentary capacity. Am J Psychiatry 114:249

9 THE RIGHT TO

TERMINATE TREATMENT

Under ordinary circumstances a patient is admitted to a psychiatric hospital either voluntarily or involuntarily, receives treatment and is discharged when his therapist and he feel he is ready for release. To imagine a patient being held any longer than necessary for treatment is difficult with the heavy pressure on state mental hospitals with an insufficient number of personnel and large patient populations. However, sometimes patients are too ill to recognize that they need treatment and may wish to terminate an experience they do not feel they require. In other instances, there may be a philosophical difference about how treatment should be conducted or how long a patient should be in a hospital for any given psychiatric condition. Under most circumstances, there are clear ways of terminating treatment. These vary from state to state and depend on the nature of the original admission, *i.e.*, voluntary or involuntary, medical or legal commitment, *et cetera.*

HYPOTHETICAL CASE EXAMPLE: R.T., a 29-year-old single, junior faculty member at a state college was admitted voluntarily to a psychiatric hospital after reporting to his psychiatrist that he felt if he were not "controlled" he would "surely kill someone." For several months he had become increasingly suspicious and distrustful and during the preceding two weeks became convinced that all his friends and relatives had been organized to extract his "inner sacred essence." He felt a mandate from God to destroy those who had formerly known him in order to save himself. On mental status examination he was grossly paranoid and had a flight of ideas.

The patient had always been suspicious and tended to isolate himself. Twice in the past year in an explosive, jealous rage he caused property damage. The first time, he began throwing dishes and glassware at a girlfriend who did not press charges. Later he smashed his own car into a tree in his yard but luckily escaped with only minor injuries. Three days after admission, he continued to feel there was a conspiracy against him. He refused medication and stated that he "must take up arms" to protect himself. He therefore decided to leave the hospital. He had packed his bags and had begun to leave when he encountered a nurse who stated he couldn't and called the director of the ward. Meanwhile, the patient contacted his lawyer who discovered it was necessary to present a written request for discharge ten days in advance in the state where the patient was hospitalized. The patient and his lawyer therefore submitted the written request. The director, disturbed by the patient's continued paranoid ideation, homicidal potential and past history of violent behavior, requested a physician outside of his own hospital to examine the patient. The other physician concurred that the patient represented a homicidal threat and filled out a medical certificate of commitment. The patient continued to protest and with his lawyer attempted to obtain his release. Throughout this time, the patient continued to refuse any therapeutic attempt, medical or psychological, to relieve his paranoid condition. After one month, he was still convinced that there was an organized plot to destroy him and that the hospital was but one link in it. Therefore the director requested the local court to commit the patient which, after the appropriate examinations and procedures, it did. At each stage, how might the patient request discharge and under what circumstances would he be granted it?

DISCUSSION

Important distinctions are made between voluntary admissions and involuntary commitment to a mental institution. The differences in the way a patient is admitted, the rights he possesses while in a mental health facility and the extent to which he may be judged incompetent to handle his personal and business affairs, particularly when he has been involuntarily committed, have been discussed. It is also true with regard to release from a mental hospital there are significant differences in the way the law treats those voluntarily admitted or those involuntarily committed. The hypothetical case clearly delineates the various ways an individual can be admitted to a mental health hospital and strongly suggests that release is closely associated with the manner of the patient's admittance. Not only is there a distinction between voluntary admission and involuntary commitment as to termination of treatment, but there are differences among the types of voluntary and involuntary admissions.

The patient in this hypothetical case originally admitted himself voluntarily to the hospital. For the most part voluntary admissions are accomplished by having the patient or guardian initiate the procedure and submit an application. When this occurs, the patient is under legal obligation to comply with certain rules on release. But, perhaps the most simple voluntary admission is one of an informal basis; the patient enters the facility without signing a statement or application for admission and is consequently entitled to leave within the day at will. Occasionally the informal voluntary admission is the only easy way to a hospitalize patient who needs care but is not suicidal or homicidal, therefore not subject to involuntary commitment in many states. This is particularly true if the patient refuses to sign an admission application. but recognizes the benefits of some hospital treatment. Because the admission is informal the patient can leave within a short time of expressing his desire to leave. There is no requirement that he give several days notice before terminating treatment in the mental institution. In this time of heightened sensitivity to the civil rights of patients and the potential abuses of unchecked control over termination of treatment, the informal admission—if possible—is probably the preferred method of admission to a mental hospital. At least ten states including New York, Pennsylvania and Connecticut have provisions in their statutes and procedures in operation for this type of admission in addition to regular voluntary admissions.

The patient who formally admits himself to a mental health institution is under legal obligation to follow specific procedures before he can leave the hospital. He is not allowed to pack his belongings and walk out of the treatment center; instead, he must submit a written request for release. In some states the written request is sufficient for immediate discharge from the hospital. In others, the patient may be required to remain in the hospital for a time before being released; this "detention" may range from 48 hours, as in the District of Columbia, to as long as 15 days in Oklahoma and a few other states. At least ten states further protect a patient from indiscriminate and unlimited hospitalization by specifying the period of time that he may be hospitalized. Voluntary hospitalization allows the patient to have an even more significant role in deciding whether treatment is to continue. In states like Virginia and Pennsylvania where voluntary admission means a 15 or 30 day maximum confinement, if the patient does not consent to maintain the therapeutic relationship, he must be released. If he agrees to continue treatment in states which provide for determinate admission he can be readmitted for another limited period of time.

Many states not only do not restrict the period of voluntary hospitalization but require that the patient agree to a certain minimum period of hospitalization before he can request release. The period of minimum hospitalization varies from as little as 15 days in some states to 60 days in others and as much as nine weeks in at least one state, Idaho. Only after the patient has remained in the hospital for a specified period can he request release through a written notice. Actual release may take as much as an additional 15 days. In all but nine or ten states, hospital authorities are not obligated to inform the patient of his right to request release under the statutes of the states. As a result a patient might admit himself voluntarily to a hospital and be unaware of the fact that he has the right to submit a written notice for release from his confinement. In effect a legally unsophisticated patient would be essentially denied his right to terminate treatment. To a great extent New York has made the most significant advance in protecting the civil rights of patients by putting into operation the mental health information service, consisting of an attorney who provides advice and legal assistance to the patients of one or more mental hospitals in the state. This service concerns itself with the full range of patient rights in treatment programs whether these patients have been voluntarily admitted or involuntarily committed to institutions.

One form of admission allowed in the statutes of many states is not exactly voluntary in that it is not brought about by the patient himself, nor is it involuntary in the sense of being a formal determination of mental illness through a judicial proceeding. "Nonprotested admission" means the patient has not initiated the admission proceeding but does not object to admission to a treatment center. If the patient, in fact, protests admission treatment cannot be accomplished through this mechanism. Once the patient has been admitted through "nonprotested admission" the procedure for terminating treatment is for the most part similar to that with voluntarily admitted patients. In any case, the patient has the right to have the issue of his release examined by the court if need be after he has indicated the desire to terminate hospitalization. In California, for example, the patient must be released within 15 days after he states in writing his desire to terminate hospitalization.

In the hypothetical case, the patient was committed on a medical certificate after he had made a written request to be discharged from the hospital. This form of involuntary commitment can be for a definite or indefinite period of time. If detention is intended as an emergency measure, the limit for keeping the patient can range from the usual five to ten days to thirty or even sixty days after which the patient must be released. Commitment to a hospital is also determinate if it is of a temporary or observational basis, for the purpose of evaluating and diagnosing as well as treating the patient. Most often this form of commitment is also for a 30 or 60 day period and may, in some states, require a hearing before a judge on the issue of the need for observational hospitalization even for that time period. If it is felt that after that period of time the patient should be kept in the hospital, a judicial proceeding is required.

Medical certification can also result in indeterminate commitment. In some states the patient may be committed for an indefinite period of time unless he demands his release in writing and takes legal steps to achieve it. In several states the decision to commit a patient indefinitely through medical certification may require the approval of a judge who will be concerned with the genuineness of the medical documents rather than with evaluating the merits of the decision to hospitalize the patient. In all the states which have medical certification proceedings, the patient is given the right either to request a judicial review of the certification or to be released within a specified time period after he gives notice of this desire.

In addition to medical certification, formal commitment proceedings exist which can involve confinement for an indefinite period. These proceedings are usually brought before a judge or jury to determine whether a patient is mentally ill and if hospitalization is essential. This decision may be based on the advice of medical experts, but it does not necessarily have to involve the opinions of medical experts. Other considerations, like the requirements for societal control and safety in specific instances, may be the decisive factors in commitment. The discretion, therefore, for determining the merits of hospitalization is left to the judge or jury. Commitment resulting from a judicial proceeding makes gaining release often more difficult for the patient, but there are ways of securing "freedom" even under these conditions.

A patient who has been involuntarily committed to a mental institution may be released from that hospital through two methods. First he may be simply discharged by the hospital authorities because they have concluded that there would be little benefit to be gained in continuing hospitalization or that the patient had in fact recovered. In many states the legal criteria used to justify an administrative discharge are quite broad. They range from allowing discharge for those patients who have recovered from their illness or were possibly never mentally ill when admitted to those patients who perhaps have not improved but are not likely to be detrimental to the public welfare or injurious to themselves (Michigan Code, 1967). For the most part an administrative discharge is complete if the patient is no longer under the surveillance of the hospital. However, most states provide that institutions can release patients but maintain custody so if necessary the patients can be returned to the hospital.

Administrative discharge depends on the opinion of medical authorities about the mental status of the patient; the patient, therefore, has no way of formally initiating an administrative discharge. But the second method of gaining his release is by bringing his case to court. The most common court proceeding available for obtaining a discharge is a *writ of habeas corpus*. This writ, emerging from the common law tradition in England, provides a way for a person who feels he is being unjustly detained and deprived of his liberty to have the issue examined in court. All the states recognize the right of mental patients to this legal recourse. In some jurisdictions the writ is limited in scope, allowing only the issue of the legality of the original detention to be examined. Where this is the policy, the question of the patient's continued confinement is never faced by the court. Therefore, if the court decides that the patient was appropriately committed and detained it will end its investigation and not even consider whether the patient should be released because he no longer needs to be hospitalized. Other courts, however, have expanded the writ to include an evaluation of the patient's mental status at the time of the habeas corpus proceeding. In these jurisdictions the court will not only determine the validity of the initial hospitalization but will also decide whether the patient needs to continue his stay in the hospital. Several states have provided specifically in their statutes that the habeas corpus proceeding consider the condition of the patient at the time of inquiry. (California Welfare and Institutions Code, 1966).

In addition to the writ of habeas corpus, the statutes of nearly 40 states also provide for another judicial discharge procedure. This proceeding may be initiated by the patient or by his family, friends and for that matter any citizen who feels that hospitalization of the patient is no longer appropriate. The distinctions between this procedure and the writ of habeas corpus are that the former always involves examining the propriety of continuing the hospitalization and often requires some medical information, such as a certificate, showing that the patient no longer needs to be hospitalized. The medical documentation of the patient's condition is often required before the judicial proceeding can be initiated. Some courts actually order their own medical examination of the patient. They determine whether the patient should be discharged on a variety of criteria from the establishment of competency, to requiring a showing that the patient's condition has "improved," to even allowing the discharge of patients who are essentially unimproved and unlikely ever to improve.

The discussion has been focused on the questions posed by the hypothetical case. Besides these there are two other questions that will be briefly explored.

1) Is it possible to qualify a discharge so that a patient can be returned to the hospital if he is unable to adjust to the community or neglects to comply with required treatment programs? Nearly all the states provide for some form of qualified release whereby the patient can be returned to the hospital without requiring a new admission or commitment proceeding if he fails to follow the conditions set out by the hospital, such as attending outpatient treatment at a clinic or returning to the hospital for follow-up. The usual period for conditional release is one year at the end of which the patient is evaluated by the hospital and a decision is made whether to discharge him or extend the conditional period. Some states allow the conditional period to be for an indefinite time at the discretion of

the hospital. The advantage of this form of release is that it releases patients sooner who really do not need to be hospitalized but at the same time do require regular followup care. In addition it provides a "testing" period during which the extent of the patient's recovery can be assessed.

2) Because of the tremendous potentiality for abusing the constitutional rights of patients, what safeguards are important for the patient? One important safeguard already discussed is the establishment of a mental health information service similar to the one in New York where patients have ready access to lawyers for advice regarding their legal rights. In addition to a mental health information service there are three other safeguards that significantly affect the rights of patients: (a) periodic review and reexamination particularly of those patients involuntarily committed to mental institutions, (b) the elimination of indefinite commitment and the requirement for periodic redetermination of the need for confinement and (c) greater use of alternatives to hospitalization, in particular the use of foster homes and day treatment programs.

REFERENCES

Brakel SJ, Rock RS (1971): The Mentally Disabled and The Law (revised ed.). Chicago, University of Chicago Press

Calif Welfare & Institutions Code, (1966) Section 5276 (Supp 1968)

Chambers DL (1972): Alternatives to civil commitment of the mentally ill: Practical guide and constitutional imperatives. Michigan Law Rev 70:1107

Chayet NL (1968): Legal neglect of the mentally ill. Am J Psychiatry 125:785

District of Columbia Code Annotated, (1967) 21–(542–546)

Guttmacher MS, Weihofen H (1952): Psychiatry and the Law. New York, WW Norton

Hitchman I, Salomon E (1966): Foster care: An alternative to hospitalization, Current Psychiatric Therapies. Edited by JH Masserman. New York, Grune & Stratton

Idaho Code Annotated, (1949) Section 66–322, (Supp 1969)

Lemert EM (1946): Legal Commitment and social control. Soc Soc Res 30:370

Lindman FT, McIntyre DM (eds) (1961): The Mentally Disabled and The Law. Chicago, University of Chicago Press

Mayer EJ (1969): Lawyer in a mental hospital. Ment Hyg 53:14

Michigan Comprehensive Laws Annotated, (1967) Section 330.35a

New York Mental Hygiene Law, (1951) (Supp 1970)

Oklahoma Revised Statutes, (1954) 43 A, Section 70–75 (Supp 1969)

Overholser W, Weihofen H (1946): Commitment of the mentally ill. Am J Psychiatry 102:762

Pennsylvania Statutes Annotated (1969) 50, Sections 4418, 4419

Rock RS (1968): Hospitalization and Discharge of the Mentally Ill. Chicago, University of Chicago Press

Ross HA (1959): Commitment of the mentally ill: problems of law and policy. Michigan Law Rev 57:945

Tancredi L, Clark D (1972): Psychiatry and the Legal Rights of Patients. Am J Psychiatry 129:104

Virginia Code Annotated, (1953) Section 37:1–98, (Supp 1968)
It is interesting to note that the authority for administrative discharge is in the vast majority of states vested in the institution. However, some states also empower a central state agency with the authority to effect administrative discharges.

PART 3

THE MENTAL HEALTH PROFESSIONAL AS WITNESS

10 THE INSANITY DEFENSE

No single aspect of forensic psychiatry has drawn as much attention as *the insanity defense*. This expression means that under certain circumstances, determined according to principles outlined in the discussion of this chapter, an individual who has committed an act that in a usual situation would be considered criminal is not held culpable by virtue of "insanity." Obviously, this is not always a simple decision and much evidence may be brought forth by both the defense and the prosecutor to support arguments pro and con. At this point a psychiatrist, in an effort toward understanding the mental illness, may be called to testify by either side. In some instances, he may be called upon to testify in the case of one of his own or former patient. At other times, he may be requested to examine a patient he has never seen before.

The determination of criminal responsibility is quite separate from the determination of an individual's ability to stand trial. In the latter instance, one is concerned with a person's actual condition at the time of his pretrial examination whereas in the former instance, one is concerned with an accused person's condition at the time of the alleged offense. A patient is generally held to be mentally unfit to stand trial for a crime in most states if he is not capable of understanding the charges made against him and if he is not able to participate in his own defense. Such a determination may in fact be quite complicated. Many seriously, psychiatrically ill individuals may be able to state quite clearly the charges made against them but actually not understand the meaning of the words they can so glibly articulate. Likewise, an individual may be quite pleasant in external appearance and be quite cooperative but because of cerebral dysfunction due to a degenerative disease, senile dementia or Huntington's chorea, for example, be quite unable to provide sufficient information and relative detail to exonerate himself with his attorney's assistance. When a patient is found unable to stand trial because of a psychiatric condition he may simply be referred for treatment and the charge dismissed if the offense is a minor one. If, however, the offense is of a more serious nature, trial may be deferred to such a time when the patient may be deemed well enough to stand trial. This obviously can lead to extreme consequences. For example, a person who is quite innocent may under the stress of having to stand trial relapse after considerable improvement as the impending trial draws near.

HYPOTHETICAL CASE EXAMPLE: I.D. is a 27-year-old black, divorced male aide at a large public city hospital. Over the course of five weeks, he became convinced that he was a special agent of God. He confided to fellow employees and to some patients, much to their dismay, that God had asked him to die for their sins just as Jesus had. I.D. interpreted several rainstorms as a sign that his "day had come." He decided to kill himself by crashing a car. He felt "the angel of the Lord" lead him to an ambulance parked at the emergency door of the hospital. The keys in the ignition confirmed to him that this was for his purposes. He closed the doors and before any attendants noticed, the ambulance was speeding down the major street of the city with siren and lights going as if on an emergency run. Coming to a turn in the road, he was convinced that a passerby was a malicious imp attempting to control him. He hit and seriously injured the pedestrian and smashed into two cars parked along the side. Amazingly, he escaped with little injury. When he was removed from the ambulance, he was crying that he had failed God because he was still alive and did not die as Christ did for man's sin, and furthermore he had not succeeded in killing the imp thus ending his reign of evil deeds. His history revealed he had been admitted to a state hospital for three months at age 18 and for six months at age 25 and was diagnosed as schizophrenic. On examination, he was delusional with racing thoughts and auditory hallucinations, but he was oriented to time, place and person.

Would he be considered able to stand trial? If so, would he be held culpable for severely injuring the pedestrian and stealing the ambulance? Would he be held responsible for the damage to the ambulance and the two parked cars?

DISCUSSION

Three broad issues are raised by this hypothetical case that will be discussed in the following order: competency to stand trial; the insanity defense and the criminal offender; and the mental patient's culpability in civil and, more specifically, tort claims. Each of these problem areas could require an extensive discussion, but only the most important issues will be highlighted.

1) What is meant by the legal concept of "competency to stand trial" and what are the consequences to the person who is considered incompetent? The requirement that an individual meet some standard of mental competence in order to stand trial is found in the provision of the United States Constitution that states that every citizen is entitled to due process of law. The interpretation of this phrase has been expanded particularly in recent years to become the basis for a variety of rights including the right to a speedy trial, the right to legal counsel and the right of the defendant to be present not only physically but also mentally to assist in his own defense at trial. In addition to the constitutional requirement for due process of law, the assurance that a defendant be mentally competent to stand trial is historically rooted in the common law tradition as adopted from the English law.

Stated succinctly, the rule for competency to stand trial consists of three specific capabilities; the defendant must be able to understand (a) the nature and object of the proceedings against him, (b) his position in relation to those proceedings and (c) be able to advise and assist in his own defense. To determine that these criteria have been satisfied it is necessary to show that the defendant understands the following features of his case: the charge that is being brought against him, and the possible outcome of the trial in terms of verdict and sentence; the persons involved with the court proceeding such as the lawyers, judge, jury and most particularly his role in the trial; the fact that the alleged act is considered by the law and most immediately the court to be a criminal offense; his legal rights such as the right to legal counsel and the Fifth Amendment protection against self-incrimination; and, the need to account for his movements in detail as well as those of others who might be involved in the case. In addition to these features, it is essential to demonstrate that the accused can cooperate and assist the counsel in preparing and presenting his case to the court. This ability to advise counsel includes helping to gather important details or facts surrounding the case as well as assisting the lawyer to challenge assertions by the prosecution and witnesses testifying against his interests.

The evaluation of the defendant's ability to stand trial is not limited to his meeting the conditions of the rule on competency. In addition to this, the psychiatrist asked to examine the accused must consider whether the accused might decompensate during the trial; the defendant might be perfectly capable of understanding the charges against him and the nature of the proceeding, yet be in such a precarious state of adjustment that he might possibly become violent or psychotic during the court proceeding. If the psychiatrist determines that the accused is unstable and may decompensate, he can reasonably recommend that he be considered incompetent to stand trial. Of course, the presence of mental illness does not in itself mean that the defendant is incompetent to stand trial. A person may be mentally ill and still meet the primary test of being able to make a rational defense and of understanding the court proceedings. Similarly a patient may have been involuntarily committed to a mental institution and still deemed competent to stand trial. At the same time, however, the accused's susceptibility to decompensation is an important consideration; the person could become acutely ill, violent and possibly suicidal during the trial.

In effect the determination of competency to stand trial is made by the court under the advice of a psychiatrist who has examined the defendant. If the court decides a defendant is unable to stand trial, the person may be either hospitalized, imprisoned or released for treatment on an out-patient basis; however, over forty states require that a person adjudged unable to stand trial must be hospitalized. The statutes of some states are not explicit as to whether the appropriate institution for detainment be a hospital or a prison. The remaining jurisdictions leave the decision up to the court, that is whether he should be hospitalized or released if the court feels that he is no potential danger to the community.

Perhaps the most distressing feature of the rule on incompetency to stand trial is that it allows indefinite commitment to a mental institution. It can be argued that hospitalization because of incompetency presumes guilt even though the accused has not been adjudged guilty on the basis of a court proceeding. This indefinite confinement ending only when the defendant is considered "competent" to stand trial is a gross violation of civil rights. The decision regarding involuntary hospitalization should be based on different criteria than that of competency to stand trial; just because a person is considered incompetent to stand trial does not mean that he should be hospitalized. Even if an individual meets both the criteria of involuntary hospitalization and incompetency to stand trial, the decision as to when he can be released from the hospital should not be based on whether he can stand trial. These are essentially separate issues and should not be merged as they are by most of the states.

In the hypothetical case of I.D. there was probably not sufficient information to decide whether the defendant would be considered incompetent to stand trial. It would appear likely, however, due to the suddenness of onset and the bizarre thinking directly related to the acts committed that he would be found incompetent, certainly during the acute phase of his illness.

2) What are the tests used to determine if a criminal act is due to insanity, and what are the consequences of such a decision for the offender? The term "insanity" is not a medical term but is instead a legal concept meaning that degree of mental disorder that relieves an offender of the criminal responsibility for his actions. The reasons for excusing persons from responsibility for their conduct is not clearly explained in the law. However, there are two compelling reasons. First, criminal culpability requires the presence of *mens rea*, or the *intent* to commit a criminal act; individuals who lack the capacity of "free will" cannot form a criminal intent and therefore do not meet this important requirement for culpability. And, second, the purposes of the criminal system—particularly those of protecting society, deterring others from criminal acts and punishing as well as rehabilitating the offender—are not served by punishing those who do not have the capacity to make a free rational choice.

At the present time there are four tests of criminal responsibility that are used by the state and federal courts to evaluate an offender suffering from a mental condition. These tests are the M'Naghten rule; the M'Naghten rule with the irresistible-impulse test; the Durham or "product" test; and the criteria for insanity promulgated by the American Law Institute's Model Penal Code, or the ALI test. Each of these tests has its advantages and shortcomings which will be examined briefly.

M'Naghten Rule

The M'Naghten test formulated in the 1840s was the first major test for determining criminal responsibility and it remains the sole test in fewer than half of the states. An additional 15 states rely on a combination of the M'Naghten rule supplemented by the irresistible-impulse test. The M'Naghten Rule states that "to establish a defense on the ground of insanity, it must be clearly proved that at the time of the committing of the act, the party accused was laboring under such a defective reason from disease of the mind as not to know the nature and quality of the act he was doing; or, if he did know it, that he did not know he was doing what was wrong." The test in effect requires showing the offender did not "know the nature and quality of the act", that the act he was doing "was wrong" and also that these conditions must be present because of a "disease of the mind." The most prevalent form of the test, however, emphasizes the requirement that the offender have the capacity of "knowing right from wrong" as this knowledge relates to the specific criminal act.

Even though the M'Naghten Rule is still used by many states it has become less popular in recent years; some states have rejected it in favor of other more advanced standards of criminal responsibility. The dissatisfaction stems from the wording of the test which many feel narrows those protected by the insanity defense. By focusing on the cognitive or intellectual faculties some argue that the test ignores other important aspects of the whole personality, most particularly the emotions and will. An insane person may know the quality and nature of an act and know it to be wrong, but because of an inability to control his emotional responses may commit the act nonetheless. In addition to the emphasis on cognitive capacities, the phrase "disease of the mind" has been narrowly interpreted by psychiatrists to refer only to psychosis, thereby eliminating a wide range of emotional disturbances.

Irresistible-Impulse Test

With the disenchantment over the M'Naghten Rule at least 15 states adopted a second test along with the M'Naghten referred to as the irresistible-impulse test. This additional test to some extent takes care of the criticism of the M'Naghten rule that it excludes for consideration those who cannot control their emotional responses. According to the irresistible-impulse rule an offender may know the difference between right and wrong but find himself under the influence of an overpowering impulse which drives him to commit the criminal act. In effect this rule recognizes that the power of free will may be impaired even though the offender intellectually recognizes the nature of his act and knows it is wrong.

The irresistible-impulse test is not relied on in any state as the only standard for criminal responsibility; instead it is a supplementary feature to the M'Naghten rule. This test and the M'Naghten rule considerably expand those who can be covered under the insanity defense. Many question whether an irresistible-impulse can exist in an individual intellectually capable of distinguishing right from wrong; others committed to the idea that the volitional element of human personality should be taken into account in the insanity defense feel that the M'Naghten test even with the irresistible-impulse component still fails to deal with the full range of those suffering from emotional problems which render them incapable of controlling their actions. Specifically, there is the criticism that the irresistible-impulse test still does not consider those under the influence of unconscious motivation operating over a long period of time, such as is seen in the "brooding" and "reflection" of the manic–depressive patient. The irresistible-impulse test implies sudden or spontaneous acts, but many courts have interpreted this test in a broader light making it applicable to emotional control of behavior in general.

Durham Test or Product Rule

The product rule was first established in a case in New Hampshire in the 1870s. The Supreme Court of that state rejected the M'Naghten test as inadequate and stipulated that the insanity defense should be used if the criminal act was the "product of mental disease" in the offender. Outside New Hampshire this rule went unnoticed as a possible standard for criminal responsibility until 1954 when the U.S. Court of Appeals in the Durham decision adopted the concept of the "product of mental disease or mental defect." In making this decision the court of appeals accepted the mind as an entity with both intellectual and emotional elements affecting the way an individual functions. By using the term "product" the Durham test encompasses both the spontaneous act under the irresistible-impulse test and an act which results from brooding and reflection over a relatively long period of time. As a result this test permits the introduction of the complete psychiatric picture of the offender for consideration by the court and jury, and consequently broadens considerably the classes of mental illness sometimes responsible for specific behaviors.

On the other hand, the effect that the Durham decision has had on expanding the scope of those covered under the insanity plea has resulted in the major criticism of the test. Many feel that the product rule permits the introduction of too much subjective information about the accused's mental state without providing any meaningful criteria for evaluating whether the defendant's behavior was impaired of emotional control or reason and therefore should be considered insane. The definitions of "mental disease or mental defect" have been left up to the court and therefore have resulted in the inclusion of a variety of conducts from narcotic addiction to general instability. No definition limits the mental conditions that should qualify under the insanity defense for the court and jury.

In light of these objections the U.S. Court of Appeals in subsequent decisions attempted to deal with the vagueness and lack of guidance of the Durham rule. In the Carter case the court addressed the causal problem of when a criminal act can be said to be the "product" of the accused's mental condition, and defined product to mean that the accused would not have committed the act in question unless he had been suffering from the mental disease, thus creating a direct relationship between the act and the mental condition. Eight years after the Durham decision, the court in the McDonald case further circumscribed the role of expert testimony by explicitly defining mental disease or defect to mean "any abnormal condition of the mind which substantially affects mental or emotional processes and behavior controls." This provided the jury with some idea of the effect a particular mental process could have on the accused's capacity to comply with the criminal law.

The major departure from the original Durham decision came from the U.S. Court of Appeals in the Brawner case decided in 1972 when the Durham test was overruled and the court adopted a test similar to that recommended by the ALI Model Penal Code. Even though the District of Columbia no longer applies the "product" test, two other jurisdictions besides New Hampshire still use this standard—Maine and the Virgin Islands.

American Law Institute's Test

This test in some respects is comparable to a combined M'Naghten rule and irresistible-impulse test, stating a person is not responsible for criminal conduct if at the time of such conduct as a result of mental disease or defect he lacks substantial capacity to *appreciate* the wrongfulness of his conduct or to *conform* his conduct to the requirements of the law. The rule also excludes "an abnormality manifested only by repeated criminal or otherwise antisocial conduct." This last condition of the rule exludes the psychopath who is defined as such simply because of repeated criminal conduct.

The ALI test is similar to the combined M'Naghten rule and irresistible-impulse test in that it merely substitutes the term "appreciate" for "know" in the M'Naghten rule and thereby encompasses emotional and intellectual capacities for "controlling" or "conforming" conduct to legal requirements. The phrase "conform" is also interpreted to include acts that result from brooding or reflection not included in the irresistible-impulse formula. It appears that the ALI test more closely connects the mental condition of the offender to the criminal act in question. This test has gained popularity over the past few years and is now accepted with minor modifications as the standard for criminal responsibility by all the federal circuit courts and at least ten states' courts. Many courts feel that this test still remains vague in terms of limiting what should be considered a mental disease or defect, and that the exact wording of the charge to the jury is not the critical issue. What is important is that the charge include three elements—a statement about the offender's intellectual abilities to decide between right and wrong, an assessment of his volition from the perspective of whether he desired to commit the crime and a consideration of his emotional capacity to control his own conduct.

Before completing this discussion it is important to note that some states allow the insanity defense to be circumvented by a doctrine of partial responsibility, allowing evidence of an abnormal condition to negate the state of mind required for various crimes, particularly the requirement of premeditation and deliberation in first degree murder. If the defendant is successful in this plea he will be convicted of a lesser crime. Also this doctrine allows evidence of mental abnormality to be introduced in order to reduce the sentence or punishment. The doctrine is used primarily in cases where there is not sufficient mental abnormality to be successful in an insanity plea, yet enough possibly to negate *mens rea*, or intent to commit a criminal act in those crimes where intent is essential for conviction. Fewer than 15 states have used this doctrine and then only infrequently, the exception being California where partial responsibility, or the Wells–Gorshen doctrine is frequently used.

If the court and jury find the offender not guilty by reason of insanity he is not likely to be set free; in fact in nearly one-third of the states he is automatically hospitalized. In a number of other states the court will decide if the individual is still mentally ill and if commitment is advisable. Should the defendant be hospitalized he would most likely not be released until he has fully recovered from his mental condition. Some states will not allow him to be released even then if there is the possibility that his mental abnormality will recur. Over half of the states leave it up to the court to decide whether the defendant can be discharged from the hospital; in other states the mental institution has the right to discharge the patient without obtaining the consent of the court. The major standards for establishing fitness for discharge are that the defendant is not likely to repeat his offense and that it is relatively safe to release him to the community.

Returning to the hypothetical case, it would be likely that the defendant would be found "not guilty by reason of insanity" for both injuring the pedestrian and stealing the ambulance, in that both the ambulance and the passerby (imp) figured prominently in his delusion. Assuming that a court were to apply the most narrow of the tests, the M'Naghten Rule, there is a strong argument that the defendant did not "know the quality and nature of the act" since he suffered from a misperception that the ambulance was sent by God and that the pedestrian was an imp. Furthermore, it could be argued that he did not "know" that what he was doing was wrong; in fact, according to the description, he thought the opposite was true. The Durham and ALI tests would probably come to the same conclusion; his act was the "product" of a mental disease or that he did not "appreciate" the "wrongfulness of his conduct."

Before discussing the third main issue of this chapter it is important to note that at least 25 states require that defendants who plead insanity must be examined by impartial experts; some of these states actually hospitalize the defendant while he is being evaluated. These compulsory mental examinations have been sharply criticized in recent years for violating the basic rights of the defendant, particularly the right against confinement without a court hearing on the reasonableness of hospitalization, and the right against self-incrimination. The Briggs Law ensures (in Massachusetts) routine psychiatric examinations for all defendants who have either been indicted for a capital offense or have been indicted (more than once) for an offense. Many other states have passed similar statutes ensuring pretrial psychiatric examinations of various classes of offenders. These statutes enable discovering underlying mental or psychiatric features which may have otherwise gone unnoticed and which should be handled differently by the court process.

3) Is the mentally ill patient susceptible to being sued on a claim for personal and property damages? The fact that an individual is mentally ill does not in itself excuse him from civil liability as in the instance of the defendant in the hypothetical case who damaged an ambulance, a pedestrian and two parked cars. He is liable to suit for these offenses despite the fact that a criminal court might find him not guilty by reason of insanity. As a general rule unless a person has been adjudged incompetent he can be sued. If he has been adjudged incompetent, notice of suit can be served on his guardian who will then represent the patient's interests in a civil trial.

REFERENCES

Allen RC, Ferster EZ, Weihofen H (1968): Mental Impairment and Legal Incompetency. New Jersey, Prentice Hall

ALI Model Penal Code, (1955) Section 4.01 (1) (Tent Draft No 4)

Bazelon DL (1974): Psychiatrists and the adversary process. Sci Am 230:18

The Briggs Law, (1932) Mass Gen Laws c 123, Section 100A, (Ter Ed)

Bromberg W (1948): Crime and The Mind: An Outline of Psychiatric Criminology. Connecticut, Greenwood Press

Carter vs United States, (1957) 252 F 2d 608 (D C Cir)

Diamond BL, Louisell D (1965): The psychiatrist as an expert witness: Some ruminations and speculations. Michigan Law Rev 63:1335

Durham vs United States, (1869) 214 F 2d 862 (DC Cir)

Fingerette H (1972): The Meaning of Criminal Insanity. Berkeley, University of California Press

Glueck S (1966): Law and Psychiatry. Baltimore, Johns Hopkins Press

Goldstein A (1970): The Insanity Defense. New Haven, Yale University Press

Gray S (1972): The insanity defense: historical development and contemporary relevance. Am Criminal Law Rev 10:559

Guttmacher G (1954): The quest for a test of criminal responsibility. Am J Psychiatry 111:428

Lindman FT, McIntyre, Jr DM (eds) (1971): The Mentally Disabled and The Law. Chicago, The University of Chicago Press

McGarry AL (1965): Competency for trial and due process via the state hospital. Am J Psychiatry 122:623

McDonald vs United States, (1962) 114 US App DC 120, 312 F 2d 847 (En banc)

M'Naghten Case (1843): House of Lords, 8 Eng Rep 718 (HL)

Morris N (1968): Psychiatry and the dangerous criminal. Southern California Law Rev 41:514

Nice RW (1968): Crime and Insanity. New York, Philosophical Library

People vs Wells, (1949) 33 Cal. 2d 330, 202 P 2d 53

People vs Gorshen, (1959) 51 Cal 2d 716, 336 P 2d 492

Robey A (1965): Criteria for competency to stand trial: A checklist for psychiatrists. Am J Psychiatry 122:616

State vs Jones, (1871) 50 NH 369, 9 Am R 242

State vs Pike, (1869) 49 NH 399, 6 Am R 533

Szasz TS (1963): Law, Liberty and Psychiatry. New York, Macmillan

United States vs Brawner, (1972) 471 F 2d 969

11 CHILD ABUSE

A painful ordeal for any psychiatric clinician is involvement in a decision to remove a child from one or both of his parents. While from an objective standpoint it might seem clear that it is in a child's best interest both physically and emotionally to be removed from a parent, seldom is this an ideal solution. Many children would probably prefer to remain with their biological parents even at tremendous peril to themselves rather than face the prospect of being reared by strangers.

Not all parents who abuse their children are mentally ill in the traditional sense. Many were abused themselves as children; others are torn with painful conflicts stemming from an unfulfilling marriage or are scarred by unresolved maturational problems. Some believe that in some instances marked economic adversity plays a precipitating role in child abuse.

A child may be in great danger if a parent is seriously mentally ill. A severely depressed mother, for instance, may feel obligated to kill her own children before she commits suicide. Sometimes a social worker, welfare worker or psychiatric clinician learns that a child is being abused and the question arises as to whether there is any way legally of inducing parents to seek psychiatric aid, of getting the abused child into treatment or of taking a maltreated child from an abusing parent and placing him in a foster home.

HYPOTHETICAL CASE EXAMPLE: C.A., a 20-year-old white, divorced mother of a three-year-old daughter, was admitted to the inpatient service of a mental health center acutely agitated and delusional with loose associations and inappropriate affect. Following an argument with her mother on the day she was admitted, she had begun to cry, pace the floor and speak incoherently.

C.A. had become pregnant during her junior year in high school and dropped out to have her baby. The father, a high school dropout who worked as a mechanic at a gas station near to her family's home, had refused to marry her. But under pressure and threats by her parents he did—only to begin to drink heavily and beat her. Remembering the pattern of her father's drinking and beatings, she felt that she had made an imprudent marriage and soon sought a divorce. C.A.'s husband felt relieved to be out of the marriage. Although a settlement had been made for her support, her ex-husband lost his job due to his drinking and she had to go on welfare. In the months following the divorce she became withdrawn and engaged in inappropriate outbursts of anger during which she would throw things at her parents or friends. Just 19 when her divorce was finalized she felt quite alone; her former friends were either in college or working at well-paid jobs that allowed them to indulge in purchasing the fashions of the day or to travel as she had always wanted. Her mother repeatedly reminded C.A. "you made your own bed and now you must lie in it." Following a particularly stressful day and one more argument she became psychotic as described earlier. Her admitting diagnosis was acute schizophrenic episode and she was placed on a phenothiazine.

During hospitalization, C.A.'s mother brought her granddaughter in to visit and the therapist noted marks on the child's body. When the child was asked where they came from, she refused to tell, but the grandmother stated that her daughter had in an angry episode punished the child by burning her with cigarettes. The patient admitted this was true, but stated she could never give up her child. The child was referred for psychiatric examination and found to be extremely anxious and tense. X-ray examination revealed healed fractures suggestive of beatings. The therapist wondered what legal course could be taken to separate this very sick mother from her abused child.

DISCUSSION

Child abuse is a most difficult problem for psychiatry and for the law to handle. Parents who commit offenses against their children could, of course, be subjected to the same treatment in the legal system as those who commit assault and battery and even murder. These crimes already exist as part of the criminal code in all states and would be just as applicable in a child abuse case as they are in injuries occurring outside of families. But for the most part existing criminal sanctions, except in the instance of very serious physical harm, are an inadequate means of dealing with child abuse as they create almost irreparable division in families. The criminal process should seldom be resorted to at the outset because it can destroy family relationships without providing other alternatives like counseling which might help to unite a family and to secure maximum benefit for the child. Removing the abused child from the family also is a high price for the child to pay; often it is better to attempt to create a moderately comfortable family than to remove the child and place him in what might appear to be an ideal environment. If it proves virtually impossible to correct a family situation then it may be necessary to resort to the legal system. All the states have provisions that allow the juvenile courts to review alleged neglect cases and if necessary to remove the child from his family. Many states also provide protective services for the abused child; efforts are made to effect changes within the family structure so that the child can remain with his parents. These services do not require a court proceeding but are usually part of a state comprehensive program for child welfare.

The hypothetical case raises the following questions involving child abuse which are of particular interest to psychiatrists and mental health workers.

1) What are the obligations of the psychiatrist and mental health worker when confronted with a highly suspicious case of child abuse? Beyond the medical obligation of assuring that the child is properly treated if the injuries are recent, the psychiatrist and mental health worker may be obligated to report instances of suspected child abuse to the legal authorities, either the presiding judge of the juvenile court or the police. Every state in the United States and the District of Columbia has some form of child-abuse reporting requirements. These requirements are contained in statutes that clearly define not only who has the obligation to report a suspicion of child abuse, but also the types of injuries that are to be reported, who should get the reports, whether or not immunity will be granted to the professional who violates professional confidence with the patient and the penalty for not reporting a suspected child abuse.

Medical doctors are required in virtually all the states to report suspicions of child abuse; nearly 20 states limit the requirement for reporting child abuse to physicians and other health care providers, like osteopaths, chiropractors and hospitals. An equal number of states place the obligation to report on nurses, a number of states include teachers and school administrators and a few states have extended the requirement to anyone who by virtue of some special relationship may have such knowledge. A few states encourage everyone to report child abuse but limit mandatory reporting to medical practitioners, because they are more likely to come into contact with child abuse and possess the most sophisticated knowledge for detecting abuse. A small number of states however do not require that the physician report a suspected case of child abuse but encourage it by granting him immunity from suits by patients who charge the physician of infracting the professional confidences inherent in the practitioner–patient relationship. In those states where reporting child abuse is mandatory for physicians or others there is often a criminal penalty if the practitioner refuses to report the event; for example, the Pennsylvania statute (1965) specifically obligates physicians, osteopaths and "any person conducting, managing or in charge of any hospital pharmacy or in charge of any ward or part of a hospital" to report instances of child abuse. If those required to report abuse fail to do so, they can be subject to a fine of $500 and/or one year in prison.

The kinds of injuries that are to be reported are often clearly described or as in the case of California (California Penal Code, 1966), "physical injury or injuries which appear to have been inflicted upon (the child) by other than accidental means by any person", are defined not in terms of seriousness of injury—gun shot wound, for example—but in terms of whether the injury could have been caused other than by accident. The physician does not have to be completely convinced, only reasonably so. He will probably base his decision on the nature of the injuries, the medical history of the patient and perhaps the likelihood of the parents abusing the child. In the hypothetical case there were the statements of the grandmother regarding the mother's treatment of the child, and physical signs, burn marks and healed fractures on x ray, giving "reasonable" grounds for suspecting child abuse.

A concern practitioners have about reporting information learned in the sanctity of the physician–patient relationship is that they will open themselves to a possible suit by the patient, though many state statutes protect the physician to varying degrees against such a suit. Some states like Pennsylvania grant unqualified immunity to practitioners; others grant immunity if the disclosure of privileged communication is done in "good faith" or without evidence of malicious intent. Even in those states not granting immunity, or if granted is conditioned on a showing of good faith or reasonable grounds, the likelihood of a practitioner being successfully sued for violating privileged communications is minimal. Probably in these circumstances the court will understand the importance of disclosing information in the legitimate interest of either the patient or other involved persons.

Interestingly, a practitioner who fails to report a suspicious case of child abuse may be civilly liable to the injured party if the state statute has a mandatory requirement for reporting such information and if it imposes criminal sanctions upon failure to do so. One could argue that by imposing criminal penalties for not reporting a case of child abuse the state is clearly singling out a class of persons who deserve special protection. Under these conditions the practitioner could also be sued for neglecting his duty to the child as defined by that state. If state regulations do not mandate that a practitioner report instances of abuse or where the statutes leave this decision up to the practitioner, the injured child would probably be unsuccessful in an action of damages against the practitioner.

2) What circumstances meet the legal requirements to justify separating a child from his parent, particularly if that parent does not give consent to such a separation? Every state acknowledges that a parent's right to keep a child can be terminated for a variety of reasons. The circumstances for separating a child from his parent include failure to support, overall neglect, cruelty, abandonment and over 40 jurisdictions include the presence of mental illness in a parent if it can be established that the parent is unable to function as a parent. In acts of direct misconduct by a parent the states vary on how they determine whether neglect or misconduct has occurred. Some states in their statutes focus on the parent or caretaker and define child neglect as existing when a parent subjects the child to cruelty or neglect. Using the criteria spelled out in some laws, it is often difficult legally to prove a parent guilty of misconduct. For child abuse to be accepted by the court a causal relationship must be demonstrated between the parent's act and the injuries suffered by the child, especially hard to do when parents are represented by lawyers. Other states focus instead on the child and claim that child abuse has occurred when a child can show the effects of being physically mistreated. In these states the court can make a decision without proof of a close relationship between injuries and specific parental misconduct. Some states are concerned with the child's environment and conclude that child abuse has occurred if a child is living in unsuitable conditions, in a filthy house without any facilities, and if it can be reasonably assumed that this is due to the depravity or cruelty of either or both parents. In states where "neglect" is defined in terms of the child's environment it is easier to establish neglect. Often simply the proof that the child has suffered several unexplained injuries suffices for the court to rule his environment unsuitable for his welfare.

The involuntary and permanent termination of a parent–child relationship because of mental illness alone may, one could argue, be usurping the rights of the natural parents; mental illness is not necessarily evidence of a lack of parental capacity. Some states require simply that the parent be "insane" or judged "incompetent" or that the condition be present for a period of years. The term "insanity" applies to a range of patients, some of whom require merely periodic outpatient visits, while others might be regressed to the point of requiring constant hospitalization. No doubt some of those described as "insane" would be unable to meet the obligations and responsibilities of parenthood, but by the same token, the largest number of those labeled "insane" would likely with minimal difficulties be able adequately to raise children. To determine "incompetency" the court must at least determine that the patient cannot deal with his business affairs, but again, that does not necessarily mean that he cannot function adequately as a parent. The modern consensus on this issue supports the notion that permanent separation is justified if the mental condition appears hopeless, incurable or might reasonably be expected to continue for a prolonged and possibly indeterminate period. The difficulty with making this decision is that modern advances in psychiatric treatment, particularly pharmacotherapy, have made possible the release of patients from care after short periods of time, patients who in the not too distant past might have required years of hospitalization. But if a mother requires three or four years of hospitalization during the child's early years and no family member can care for the child there might be justification in separating the two. Similarly, when a patient refuses treatment or when the prognosis for recovery is poor, termination of parental capacity may be the only recourse.

In the preceding hypothetical case justification for termination of the parent–child relationship does not have to involve the issue of mental illness. There is sufficient evidence, particularly the testimony of the grandmother, to convince a court that the parent had significantly abused her child. The issue of mental illness might become important should someone decide to initiate criminal charges against the parent as the argument might be made that the psychotic parent should not be held criminally responsible for these abuses. With regard to termination of the relationship the mental illness of the parent would probably have little effect on the decision to separate the child from the parent, especially since the x rays disclosed that abuses were not limited to this episode, precluding the assumption that abuse would end once the patient recuperated from her acute psychotic condition.

3) Can a mentally ill patient have the capacity to consent to separation from her child, and how would such a capacity be determined? Under ordinary circumstances parents may not without their consent be deprived of custody of their children. We have already discussed the exceptions to this as in the case of flagrant misconduct towards children or serious mental illness when children may be taken away from their parent by a court decision. When the parents are separated or divorced the court may favor one parent over the other for custody of children without requiring consent basing this decision on significantly less powerful grounds than child abuse. In these cases there is a trend toward using an affirmative test, such as "what is in the best interests of the child" to justify separation of a child from a parent rather than the far more difficult test to prove child abuse.

When consent is required for an agreement to be valid, the issue of mental incompetency is most important. If a patient can allege years after she has consented to the termination of her relationship with a child and years after that child has been adopted by other "parents" that she was not mentally competent at the time to understand the nature of the agreement to which she had consented, the court may allow her to revoke her earlier consent. This could be extremely disruptive and damaging to the child and cruel for the adoptive parent who in good faith adopted the child thinking that the natural parent had given full and valid consent.

There have been only a few cases of this nature in determining when a mentally ill parent should be considered incompetent. The test recommended and used in a few of these court cases was similar to that used for determining a mentally ill patient's competency to engage in a business transaction such as signing a contract.

That test is whether the patient understands the "nature and quality" of the transaction or agreement. No test has received widespread acceptance and the law is still exploring ways to assure the rights of the mentally ill parent and at the same time prevent the hardship to all parties involved when years later a parent is able to revoke a consent to termination of his relationship with a child or to adoption. Devices being considered and used range from the appointment of guardians to safeguard the mentally ill patient's rights to the appointment of legal counsel while consent to parental separation is being considered. Perhaps the law should require a formal proceeding of some sort when consent is being executed; for example, it might be best to require that consent be executed before a government official or social worker. There does not exist at the present time any clear cut test for determining when a patient may be considered capable of consenting to separation from his child.

REFERENCES

Allen RC, Ferster EZ, Weihofen H (1968): Mental Impairment and Legal Incompetency. New Jersey, Prentice Hall

Bakan D (1971): Slaughter of The Innocents. San Francisco, Jossey-Bass

Benedek EP (1972): Child custody laws: Their psychiatric implications. Am J Psychiatry 129:102

Brakel SJ, Rock RS (1971): The Mentally Disabled and The Law (revised ed). Chicago, University of Chicago Press

California Penal Code, (1966) Section 11161.5 (Supp)

Comment (1961): Revocation of parental consent to adoption: Legal doctrine and social policy. University Chicago Law Rev 28:564

Davidson HA (1965): Forensic Psychiatry. New York, Ronald Press

Helfer RE, Kempe CH (eds) (1968): The Battered Child. Chicago, University of Chicago Press

Kempe CH, Helfer RE (1972): Helping The Battered Child and His Family. Philadelphia, JB Lippincott

Note (1952): Attacks on adoption decrees by natural parents to regain custody. Yale Law J 61:591

Note (1955): Due process rights of mentally ill parents in nonconsensual adoptions. Indiana Law J 30:431

Pennsylvania Statute Annotated, (1965) tit 18 Section 4330 (Supp)

Ritz J (1957) Termination of parental rights to free child for adoption. New York University Law Rev 32:579

Robitscher JB (1966): Pursuit of Agreement, Psychiatry and The Law. Philadelphia, JB Lippincott

Westman J (1971): The psychiatrist and child custody contests. Am J Psychiatry 127:1687

12 SEXUAL DEVIANCY

The traditional concept of sexual deviancy is undergoing revision in contemporary society. Just as in the case of the use of mild psychedelic agents among adults (such as *cannabis sativa*, or marijuana), it appears that many of the medicolegal injunctions against certain behaviors among consenting adults have more of a politicoeconomic basis than an actual ethical concern for an individual's health or the deterioration of his moral fiber. The laws affecting sexual behavior appear ludicrous—as do those imposing severe penalties on those who smoke marijuana —in contrast to the widespread toleration of the use of alcohol among adults, a behavior which results in physical harm, frequently causing the breakup of a family through economic loss as well as psychological injury, and often harm or death to others in car accidents. Neither sexual deviancy nor marijuana consumption produces comparable ruin. Today we are tolerating greater sexual expression; the laws against fornication, adultery, contraception and homosexuality served roles other than the protection of the "morality of society." Indiscriminate sexual behavior in the past led to the massive spread of veneral disease and unwanted pregnancies. Today with antibiotics and effective contraceptives, adults can elect to express themselves sexually without fear of disease or pregnancy. Furthermore, economic prerogatives have changed. Before agribusiness a large family was needed to harvest crops and to provide economic security for an individual in his senior years. These are still presented as reasons for the failure of people to adopt effective family planning in some nontechnological nations. A wife was indispensable in the home to make meals, bake bread, sew clothes *et cetera*. Today with "zero population growth" (ZPG) as an ethic, a small family has become the goal and women are freed by technological advances from the need to be role-stereotyped into "homemaking" and "motherhood." Contraception, abortion, adultery, fornication, homosexuality, bisexuality and masturbation are more accepted.

At the turn of the century people believed masturbation, politely referred to as self-abuse, would lead to all sorts of physical and psychiatric maladies. The importance of restricting sexual release directly to procreative activities so as to encourage men and women to marry and have large families was not publicly acknowledged. Fifteen years ago abortion was in most cases illegal and even a mortal sin in the Roman Catholic Church; for a woman to desire an abortion was to reject her role as "mother" or "woman." Today a physician who denies a woman an abortion is in many places accused of denying her the right to decide what to do with her own body. Comparably, in the growing freedom of sexual expression authenticity will be the factor for deciding whether two adults give their bodies to each other.

Medicine, particularly psychoanalysis, has assumed religion's role as keeper of the traditional *mores*, and law in collusion with medicine has provided the sanctions against nonconforming sexual behavior. In addition to the very real social and medical issues that ethically precluded indiscriminate sexual behavior in the past, dynamic theories of "hatred," "fear" or "anxiety" were used to explain lack of commitment to one person or to a particular sex and also to control promiscuous behavior. Today a critical reassessment of these older psychiatric postures is taking place and, as with contraception, abortion and masturbation, some behaviors labeled sexually "deviant" among consenting healthy adults will be suddenly seen as "rights," "privileges" or just "doing one's own thing."

Certain behaviors however seem to be injurious to other individuals and therefore are ethically unacceptable and must be discouraged in a humanitarian society. One of these obviously would be sexual involvement of adults with children who are not mature enough to know the implications of their actions or have not yet acquired the ability rationally to choose to become involved sexually in any given way. Sexual abuse of children in general is labeled *pederosis;* pederasty is a term more explicitly referring to sodomy and intercourse between a man and a boy.

HYPOTHETICAL CASE EXAMPLE: S.D., a 55-year-old white, agnostic, married businessman was in treatment for a mild depression with a private psychiatrist in the Midwest. During the course of treatment he was arrested on the complaint of a neighbor who found him undressing his seven-year-old daughter and fondling her genitals. S.D. cried and readily admitted his guilt. His wife was sympathetic and supportive despite his angry neighbor's efforts to get "the sex pervert off the streets." She asked his psychiatrist about the laws governing sexual molestation of children and what role psychiatry, if any, would play in her husband's disposition?

DISCUSSION

In the past those individuals who were found guilty of sexually molesting a child or of other "sex" crimes were subjected to the criminal process and if found guilty were often imprisoned for long periods of time. Some who were seriously mentally ill were able to successfully employ the traditional tests of insanity, such as the M'Naghten rule, to avoid being held criminally responsible for their acts, but many had no recourse other than the criminal system even though it had been known for a long time that many sex offenders had some degree of mental impairment.

The first "sexual" psychopath statutes were enacted in the late 1930s in Illinois and Michigan. These statutes permit involuntary hospitalization rather than imprisonment of mentally disabled persons who repeatedly commit antisocial or criminal acts. Their scope encompasses more than just sexual deviation, but are primarily used in connection with sexual conduct. Since the passage of the first acts 26 states have enacted similar legislative "safeguards" of psychopaths. The under-lying theory behind the passage of such legislation is that incarceration neither deters such acts in the future nor does it assure rehabilitation so that an offender could be returned to the community with reasonable certainty that he would not repeat the offense. In addition the legislation reflects confidence in the role that psychiatry can have in detecting potential sexual offenders and in treating them to improve the mental condition that is responsible for their "inappropriate" behavior. The most frequent psychiatric conditions associated with sexual offenses are mental retardation, psychosis, psychoneurosis, alcoholism and psychopathic behavior. Some of these conditions, particularly mental retardation and psy-chopathic behavior, are probably minimally affected by psychiatric intervention. But involuntary commitment with its potentiality for indeterminate confinement can more effectively serve the same role as imprisonment in protecting society from offenders. On the other hand, psychosis, psychoneurosis and, to a lesser extent, alcoholism can be readily benefited by medical or psychiatric treatment.

Even though treatment may be superior to imprisonment, the law also has to justify its handling of a certain class of criminals differently than those who are channeled through the criminal process. It could properly be argued that all criminals to some extent could benefit from psychiatric treatment and why, there-fore, should sexual psychopaths be handled specially? The states that provide for treatment of sexual psychopaths answer this question by claiming that the sexual psychopath is one who is unable to control his sexual acts and therefore is not legally responsible for his behavior; but this perception is inconsistent. First, why should psychopathic behavior in general, an inability to control antisocial or crimi-nal conduct, be treated differently than sexual psychopathy? Furthermore, the distinction between the sexual psychopath and the legally insane is muddied; for example the Alabama statute (1958) specifically sees the sexual psychopath as evidencing behavior that is just short of legal insanity, but criminally irresponsible nonetheless: ". . . (person) suffering from a mental disorder but is not mentally ill or feebleminded to an extent making him criminally irresponsible for his acts, such mental disorder . . . is hereby declared to be a criminal sexual psychopathic person." Despite these inconsistencies, the majority of states make this distinction so that only a very few, like Maryland and Connecticut, have expanded the group of criminally irresponsible psychopaths to the general class of those who are unable to control antisocial or criminal behavior as shown by repeated criminal activity.

The sexual psychopath statutes stipulate that the offender who claims that he should be evaluated under this legislation is to be examined by two or more court-appointed psychiatrists, or in some states physicians, before the hearing is held on the criminal act. In some states the defendant may be examined briefly by the physicians without the requirement that he be hospitalized; other states however may require that the offender by hospitalized for a varying period of observation, usually 30 days, but in at least one state as long as 120 days. Often if the psychiatrist concludes that the defendant is a sexual psychopath he does not have to return to the court but instead is placed in a treatment program. Some states require a separate hearing before a judge or jury to determine on the basis of the medical reports if the offender is a sexual psychopath according to the criteria of the statutes. At this hearing the defendant has the right to have his attorney present to represent his interests.

If at the hearing the defendant is found to be a sexual psychopath, he is placed in an appropriate treatment program for the mental abnormality that is responsible for his conduct. Several states provide that once he has successfully completed the treatment program he can be released. Others may not consider the treatment time as a substitute for fulfilling the sentence for the original crime.

In the hypothetical case the depressed patient would likely be treated as a sexual psychopath if he is in a state that has a statute which provides for hospitalization rather than imprisonment. If, in fact, he is under the rules of a state that does not recognize the special status of the sexual psychopath, he may be found guilty of the sexual act in a court case and sentenced to a period of imprisonment. The psychiatric information about the offender does not suggest that he would qualify for consideration under any of the four major tests for legal insanity—the M'Naghten Rule, the irresistible-impulse test, the Durham rule and the American Law Institutes Model Penal Code as discussed in Chapter 10.

In addition to the major issue regarding the legal consequences of sexual "psychopathic" behavior, this case raises two broader questions.

1) What are the dangers of using the medical model, or more specifically psychiatry, rather than the traditional criminal system for handling the sexual psychopath as well as those who may be classified as general psychopathic personalities? In his book *The Right to Be Different* Kittrie (1971) reveals the increasing use of medicine in the disposition of criminals and the implications that this trend has on safeguarding of the constitutional rights of these criminals. A few states have already expanded the role of the medical model making it applicable to all psychopaths not just sexual offenders. For illustration, the Maryland statute (1967) is very broad in its scope and allows the introduction of much psychiatric information into the criminal field. It defines a psychopath or "defective delinquent" as one who "(demonstrates) . . . persistent aggravated antisocial or criminal behavior, evidences a propensity toward criminal activity, and who is found to have either such intellectual deficiency or emotional unbalance, or both, as to clearly demonstrate an actual danger to society so as to require . . . confinement and treatment . . ." The sweep of this and similar statutes is so broad that under certain conditions nearly all criminal offenders could be found within its reach.

The dangers in using the treatment model rather than the criminal system concern the extent to which important constitutionally defined rights of the criminal can be circumvented in the treatment model. The laws involving involuntary commitment for treatment are civil laws and consequently important rights like the right against self-incrimination, the right of confrontation on the substantive issue of psychopathy and the right to counsel have often been denied during sexual psychopath proceedings. In criminal proceedings these rights, particularly the right to notice and a hearing on the accusation against the presumed offender, are constitutionally essential. When a determination of sexual psychopathy is to be made after a defendant is convicted of a criminal act (postconviction) the U.S. Supreme Court recently held that the offender has a right to a hearing on the issue of sex psychopathy and other rights of due process of law despite the fact that it might be a civil proceeding (Specht vs Patterson, 1967). But over a third of the states decide the issue of sexual psychopathy before an offender is convicted of a crime (preconviction) and in these cases important constitutional rights governing criminal proceedings do not necessarily apply.

With the danger of being denied important rights there is the possibility that the offender once designated a psychopath may be hospitalized indefinitely. Conceivably a person could commit a relatively innocuous act like peeping in windows and find himself committed for a much longer period of time in a hospital than he would have been in a prison under a reasonable sentence. Augmenting this possibility is the growing doubt that meaningful treatment exists successfully to cure the psychopath and to justify dealing with him differently than with others who commit socially unacceptable acts. There doesn't seem to be any solid evidence that treatment programs affect in any appreciable way the prevention of additional offenses by the psychopath. Also, many hospitals don't bother to provide any treatment for offenders who have been involuntarily committed. The U.S. Courts of Appeals for the District of Columbia in 1966 (Millard vs Cameron) extended the right of treatment concept to those committed for sexual psychopathy. Nonetheless, many jurisdictions neither recognize this right nor inquire as to the existence and use of treatment programs. As an earlier chapter on involuntary commitment suggests, there should be continuous periodic review of the reasons for confinement and evaluation of treatment facilities.

2) Thus far, the discussion has centered on sexual acts that affect others; what are the legal proscriptions, if any, against sexual deviancy involving consenting adults? In the late 1950s the Wolfenden Report was published in England which proclaimed that the function of the law is not to interfere in the private lives of citizens for the purpose of imposing particular patterns of behavior unless such "deviant" activities are injurious to others. The authors of the report recognized that opinions as to what is offensive and injurious to society differ greatly and are based on a variety of moral cultural standards. As a result, the report specifically recommended that laws against homosexual behavior between consenting adults be repealed since such behavior is not harmful to others. The Wolfenden Report sparked a series of debates whether any behavior among consenting adults in privacy offends the common good. The resolution of much discussion was the passage in England of the Sexual Offenses Act of 1967 which in effect repealed all criminal penalties for homosexual acts between consenting adults in privacy.

The American laws have nonetheless remained prohibitive of activities such as sodomy, homosexuality and even fornication among consenting adults. However there seems to be a trend toward liberalization of these laws in recent years; at least eight states have repealed their statutes that prohibited sodomy between consenting adults and similarly no longer penalize homosexual relationships. States like Connecticut, Hawaii, Illinois and Oregon no longer have laws against sodomy and interestingly, the American Law Institute's revised 1962 Model Penal Code contains no provision making homosexual conduct between consenting adults a criminal offense. The code does of course continue strongly to prohibit sexual acts between adults and children or those that involve coercion with threats of serious bodily harm or death. Even some municipalities have liberalized their laws on consensual sexual acts; most conspicuously, Washington D.C. passed in November 1973 the Human Rights Law (Title 34) prohibiting discrimination in public and private employment, housing and use of public accommodations on the basis of homosexuality.

The reason for statutes against homosexual behavior has often been presented as the need to deter others from engaging in such conduct. The Wolfenden Report, however, questioned the validity of that statement for it found no evidence of an increase in the prevalence of such behavior in countries where homosexuality and other forms of sexual deviance involving consenting adults are condoned. Furthermore, the function of rehabilitating those who break laws is definitely not served where sexual deviants are concerned since imprisoning the deviant only places him in an environment where alternative sexual conduct is rampant. Certainly the most important argument against the statutes prohibiting any nonharmful sexual behavior between consenting adults in privacy is that the emphasis morally and even legally should be on the authenticity of the relationship between two people rather than the way in which it is manifested. Morality should be more concerned with fraud and deceit in interpersonal relationships rather than the means by which individuals express friendship and love. Where law is concerned, the emphasis should be on preventing harm to others and preserving the sanctity of privacy whenever possible.

REFERENCES

Alabama Code, (1958) 15 Section 434 (S7pp 1967)

Brakel SJ, Rock RS (1971): The Mentally Disabled and the Law (revised ed). Chicago, University of Chicago Press

Chambliss WJ (1969): Crime and the Legal Process. New York, McGraw Hill

Committee on Homosexual Offenses and Prostitution (1963): The Wolfenden Report. New York, Stein & Day

Davidson HA (1965): Forensic Psychiatry. New York, Ronald Press

Devlin P (1965): The Enforcement of Morals. London, Oxford University Press

Fisher RG (1967–68): The legacy of Freud—a dilemma for handling offenders in general and sex offenders in particular. University Colorado Law Rev. 40:242

Goffman E (1963): Stigma—Notes on the Management of Spoiled Identity. New Jersey, Prentice Hall

Harris RN (1967): Private consensual adult behavior: The requirement of harm to others in the enforcement of morality. UCLA Law Rev 14:581

Hart HLA (1963): Law, Liberty and Morality. California, Stanford University Press

Human Rights Law, (1973) (Washington, DC), Title 34

Kittrie N (1971): The Right to be Different: Deviance and Enforced Therapy. Baltimore, Johns Hopkins Press

Maryland Annotated Code, (1967) 31 B, Section 5

Millard vs Cameron, (1966) 373 F 2d 468, (DC Cir)

Model Penal Code, (1955) Section 207.5, Comment (Tent draft No 4) Model Penal Code, (1962) Sections 213.2–213.4

Pearson vs Probate Court, (1940) 309 US 270 Minnesota case where Supreme Court of United States upheld psychopathy laws.

Sexual Offenses Act, (1967) Eliz, II Pt II C 60

Slaby AE, Tancredi LR (In Press): Collusion for Conformity. New York, Jason Aronson

Slovenko R (ed) (1965): Sexual Behavior and the Law. Illinois, Charles C. Thomas

Specht vs Patterson, (1967) 386 US 605

13 DRUG ADDICTION

The treatment of drug addiction is difficult and an activity not relished by many psychiatric clinicians, who find varying degrees of success with existing treatment programs. Sometimes less orthodox approaches involving former addicts in therapeutic roles have been most successful. While there may be sympathy with the poverty and lack of social or educational opportunity that appears to provide the milieu for the development of opiate or other drug addictives, one cannot overlook the crimes that are associated with the desperate search for funds so that more drugs can be procured (muggings, burglaries). A psychiatric clinician often encounters individuals either in search of drugs to prevent withdrawal or in the hospital for the purpose of achieving withdrawal. In addition he may treat a patient who has been arrested for the use of, possession of or sale of narcotics and wonder about the laws in their specific state.

HYPOTHETICAL CASE EXAMPLE: D.A., a 33-year-old black, Protestant, divorced male was being treated in group therapy at a mental health center for depression due to an inability to hold a job for a sustained period of time. The therapist did not feel D.A. was actively involved in the group and at times was concerned over his patient's inability to stay awake during the group sessions, but he was gratified by the fact though that D.A. rarely missed the group meetings.

After one of the sessions when D.A.'s absence was quite noticeable, the group therapist received a phone call from a public defender who informed him that D.A. had been arrested in a raid in which he was found possessing narcotics. The group therapist wondered what the laws were regulating the use of narcotics in the state, and particularly whether the fact that D.A. was undergoing treatment for a mental disorder would influence his ultimate disposition in the criminal system (*e.g.*, jail, release or bond and psychiatric treatment).

DISCUSSION

This illustration raises several interesting questions especially in the light of a recent Supreme Court decision that attempted to exclude from legal control the "state" of being an addict. Before dealing with the issues, however, it is important to show once again the possible application of the insanity defense to criminal behavior. If it can be shown that the patient in this hypothetical case meets the criteria of one of the tests for legal insanity, *i.e.*, M'Naghten, Durham, ALI formula, *et cetera*, then he would probably not be held responsible for any criminal act and instead would be placed in a treatment program. In the absence of such a defense the offender would be subject to the criminal system on a federal, state or local basis.

The federal control of drug usage began officially in 1914 with the Harrison Narcotic Act which formed the basic federal position on drugs for nearly 60 years. In effect this act mildly regulated various narcotics by requiring registration and record. Interestingly, marijuana was not included under its control and except for minimal federal regulation under the earlier Pure Food and Drug Act of 1906 marijuana was not regulated federally until 1937. The Narcotic Control Act of 1956 created severe penalties for drug abuse, increasing the minimum and maximum penalties for all drug offenses. A first conviction could receive a penalty of from two to ten years and up to 40 years for succeeding convictions. There was also added a separate penalty of 10 to 40 years for those who sold or distributed drugs to a minor and the possibility of life imprisonment and even death if the drug sold were heroin. The next major act dealing specifically with penalties for drug possession and use was the Comprehensive Drug Abuse Prevention and Control Act passed in the 1970s. This act attempted to integrate everything congress had enacted from the Harrison Act through the Marijuana Tax Act of 1936 and and the 1956 Narcotic Control Act into one "comprehensive" act. This act removed the very strong mandatory minimums of the 1956 Narcotics Control Act for most classes of drug usage. These mandatory minimums were harsh; for example the conviction for subsequent offenses could have brought a sentence as high as 40 years, but more significantly it had to be at least ten years. In addition to federal regulations there are state and local laws. Over forty states including the District of Columbia have passed a Uniform State Narcotics Law which attempts to control illicit small-time traffic of drugs. These laws also control the behavior associated with drugs from possession, use of and sale of narcotics to any crimes that may be committed under the influence of drugs. Local laws in cities (Chicago and other municipalities) also exist attempting to control the traffic of drugs by punishing possession, sale, *et cetera*. State laws may be quite severe, though less than comparable federal penalties. For example in Ohio the mere possession of drugs for sale in the future (inferred by amount in possession) may be punishable by a fine of up to $10,000 and imprisonment for from two to fifteen years. As a rule it is easier to convict drug addicts in state and local courts because the rules of evidence— what information can be admitted at a trial—are less strict that in a federal court.

In addition to discussing the laws which regulate usage of drugs, four other questions emerge which will be briefly discussed.

1) Is drug addiction a disease, and what are the legal implications of classifying it as such? The Supreme Court of the United States recognized in the Linder case early in the mid-1920s that narcotic addiction is a disease and addicts are sick

persons. However the court did not at that time prohibit the conviction of persons for being addicts *per se*. It was not until the early 1960s that the Supreme Court attempted to deal with that specific issue. In the Robinson case the court explicitly held that addiction is not only an illness but that it would be violating the safeguards in the Bill of Rights to punish individuals for being addicts. The state of California had a statute making it a crime to "be addicted to the use of narcotics." Robinson had been found guilty of this offense and according to law was sentenced to serve a minimum of 90 days in confinement for his condition. The Supreme Court held that addiction without an overt criminal act is merely a status or condition similar to being mentally ill or being afflicted with a venereal disease, and therefore should not be criminally punished. In reaching this decision the court did not rely on establishing that the addict lacked free will or the volition to abide by societal demands as it does for an insanity defense, but rather it attempted to characterize the condition itself as an illness.

The decision in the Robinson case is limited to the distinction that addiction in itself should not be considered a crime. This case does not affect the punishment of those charged with related crimes such as possession of narcotics, use of drugs or sale and transportation of narcotics across state lines. These offenses as well as those committed while under the influence of drugs have not been decriminalized, though an attempt was made a year after the Robinson decision to extend decriminalization to these offenses. The argument in this case was that drug addicts seek drugs to maintain their mental and physical balance and that this is all part of the disease process; consequently the possession and use of narcotics is merely a feature of the overall illness and should not be punished. The U. S. Courts of Appeals for the District of Columbia upheld the conviction; the narrow interpretation of the Robinson case remains for all jurisdictions (Horton vs United States, 1962).

2) Is a therapist obligated under the doctrine of privileged communication to refrain from testifying that his patient is engaged in any illegal activity related to narcotics? The doctrine of privileged communication is recognized in over 30 states and essentially it prevents a physician from disclosing information obtained during the course of medical treatment during litigation or a court proceeding. This rule is usually applied to physicians, but a growing number of states like New York have extended the obligation to any person involved in the care of patients —psychologists, nurses, social workers, *et cetera*.

However, the right of the patient to require that personal information be kept confidential is not an unrestricted right, for some states wave the privileged communication rule when there is strong public policy in favor of disclosing patient information. One such situation would be narcotics addiction, especially when where possession, selling and transporting of drugs are involved. Narcotics addiction is rarely a personal, private act and it inevitably affects others in society— mostly the young and poor of the city ghettoes. A major social policy would be to try to discover the links in a chain of narcotics peddling; consequently most states waive the privileged communication rule in the case of narcotics addiction. Although the therapist may not be legally required to report a patient who possesses or uses narcotics, he may be compelled to testify in court.

3) If addiction to a drug is a disease state, are drug addicts subject to involuntary commitment? Over 30 states have provisions in their mental illness laws for commitment of those suffering from narcotics addiction. An addict who is being involuntarily committed is often given a judicial hearing and confined to a state

mental institution if there are no specialized facilities available. If facilities are available that deal specifically with drug problems, the addict may be committed there until he is considered cured or sufficiently improved.

One of the difficulties of committing drug addicts is that the state statutes for the most part do not clearly define that level of addiction necessary for involuntary commitment; some states rely strictly on a medical definition of an addict, *i.e.*, one who has habitually used a drug to the point of developing a tolerance for the drug and there is not a health need that he be on such medication. Others define an addict in terms of societal safety; for example, the Oregon statute states that a person can be committed who habitually uses a habit-forming drug and who as a result endangers the public health, safety or morals. Maryland in contrast defines an addict as one who uses specific drugs such as cocaine or morphine to the degree that he is deprived of "reasonable self-control."

Involuntary commitment of the mentally ill is similar to the drug addict, particularly in that he may lose important rights when he has been involuntarily committed. This could include the right to form contracts, as well as the right to conduct other private, personal affairs. In addition the drug addict, since he has most likely been committed through a judicial proceeding, finds it very difficult to terminate his commitment. The court may have the final word in deciding whether the addict should be released from the hospital. An addict may be released in a relatively short time if he has entered a suitable program that specializes in withdrawing addicts from narcotics; if because of limited facilities he finds himself in a state mental institution he may be confined for an inappropriately long period of time.

4) Are the penalties against the use of marijuana similar to those against the use of narcotics or other drugs? It was not until the Marijuana Tax Act in 1937 that marijuana was associated with other narcotics. In subsequent legislation like the Narcotics Control Act of 1956 marijuana contined to be included with the other "habit-forming" drugs like heroin and morphine. However, the attitude toward strong controls of marijuana and other drugs with legal sanctions has shifted toward greater reliance on the medical profession for drug treatment. This shift became most pronounced in the 1960s. The White House Conference on Narcotic and Drug Abuse in its report in 1962 stated that there was only minimal association between marijuana and criminal activity, that the drug was not truly addicting like heroin and the opiates and that in general the hazards of marijuana had been exaggerated. The President's Advisory Commission on Narcotics and Drug Abuse in 1963 even further distinguished marijuana from addicting drugs. This commission took issue with the idea that high penalties, mandatory minimum fines and jail terms effectively deterred drug abuse and further supported the growing belief that marijuana does not induce physical dependence.

Finally in 1967 The Marijuana Tax Act came under considerable attack in the Report of the Commission on Law Enforcement and Administration of Justice; the commission suggested that the act was ineffective since only a few persons were ever registered under it. Furthermore, it felt it was an inappropriate act because it equated the usage of marijuana with that of the opiates. The commission felt that the effects of marijuana were completely different from other narcotic addicting drugs. This report highlighted a series of commentaries that called into question previously held notions that marijuana usage was equivalent to narcotic addiction. To a great extent this new view of marijuana was generated by the realization that drug addiction in general did not necessarily cause criminal behavior and marijuana in particular was not correlated with a statistically significant increase in crime nor did marijuana seem to have any of the physical or mental side effects that characterized other addictive drugs.

Although the federal position on drug abuse and marijuana usage has not changed appreciably in recent years, there have been several interesting developments regarding the state laws on drug abuse. Of the 50 states over 30 recommend a conditional discharge for a first offense of possession of marijuana. Oregon has significantly altered its statute. In an act which became law in late 1973, criminal penalties for possession of marijuana were reduced considerably for a first offense; if a marijuana user is found with less than one ounce of marijuana in his first offense the legal sanction is comparable to a traffic violation with a maximum fine of $100 and no jail sentence. Even Texas, which at one time had the most severe law in the country, has significantly mitigated its position to the point of making private possession of a small amount of marijuana equivalent to a minor misdemeanor. At the present time Rhode Island is the only state that continues to consider a first offense of marijuana possession a felony offense.

In addition to the significant changes occurring in state legislations in 1972 there was a very important case decided by the Supreme Court of Hawaii; a majority of that court held the private possession of marijuana cannot be constitutionally considered a crime. The reasoning was that until legitimate, medical research proves otherwise, it is far more harmful to designate as criminal an activity involving a large proportion of the population who are otherwise considered law abiding citizens, and that there is no benefit in classifying marijuana as a narcotic. The presiding judge went on to state that there appears to be no logical reason for society to control this act at the present time (State vs. Kantner, 1972). Other cases involving marijuana usage are being considered by the courts at the present time and the results may reveal a more enlightened attitude toward this issue.

REFERENCES

Aronowitz R (1967): Civil commitment of narcotic addicts. Columbia Law Rev 67: 405

California Welfare & Institution Code, (1966) Sect. 3100 (West)

Chun G (1971): Marijuana: A realistic approach. Calif Med 114:7–13

Disclosure of confidential information. (1971) JAMA 216:385

Frankel M (1966): Narcotic addiction, criminal responsibility and civil commitment. Utah Law Rev 581

Horton vs US, (1963) 317 F 2d 595 (DC Cir)

King R (1972): The Drug Hang-Up: America's Fifty-Year Folly. New York, WW Norton

Kittrie N (1971): The Right to be Different: Deviance and Enforced Therapy. Baltimore, Johns Hopkins Press

Linder vs United States, (1925) 268 US 5

The Marijuana Tax Act, (1937) PL 75–238, 50 Stat 551

Maryland Code Annotated, (1966) Art 16 and 43 (Repl vol)

Maurer DW, Vogel VH (1967): Narcotics and Narcotic Addiction. Illinois, Charles C Thomas

Morse HN (1971): The tort liability of the psychiatrist. Baylor Law Rev 19:208

Musto DF (1973): The American Disease: Origins of Narcotic Control. New Haven, Yale University Press

National Commission on Marijuana and Drug Abuse (1973): Reports of the National Commission on Marijuana and Drug Abuse. Washington, DC, Government Printing Office

Neill WC (1970): Legal aspects of drug abuse. Cleveland State Law Rev 19:461

New York Civil Rights Law, (1972) Act 45, Sections 4501, 4507, 4508

New York Mental Hygiene Law, (1966) Sections 200–217 (McKinney Supp)

NORML (October 10, 1973), Statement on Impending Civil Suit.

Note (1974): Developments in the law—Civil commitment of the mentally ill. Harvard Law Rev 87:1190

Ohio Revised Code, (1964) Sections 371909 and 3719.99 (C)

Oregon Revised Statute (1957) 475.610 (1)

President's Advisory Commission on Narcotics and Drug Abuse, Final Report. (1963) Washington, DC, Government Printing Office.

President's Commission on Law Enforcement and Administration of Justice, Task Force Report (1967): Narcotic and Drug Abuse. Washington, DC, Government Printing Office

Proceedings of the White House Conference on Narcotics and Drug Abuse, Final Report. (1962) Washington DC, Government Printing Office

Robinson vs California, (1962) 370 US 660

Slaby AE, Tancredi LR (In Press): Collusion for Conformity. New York, Jason Aronson

State vs Kantner, (1972) 53 Haw 327, 493 P 2d 306 cert denied, 409 US 948

14 ALCOHOLISM

Patients having problems with alcohol require a mental health clinician to have some familiarity with the laws of his state concerning alcoholism, the question of criminal responsibility of intoxicated patients as well as the laws regarding commitment of individuals with alcohol problems for treatment. Is a patient under the influence of alcohol legally culpable if he kills someone or is violent toward person or property? How would the courts be likely to handle this issue? Can a clinician who sees a patient repeatedly suffering from intoxication, severe nutritional deficiency and overall physical debilitation commit him for a treatment program? Do the courts ever legally commit to a mental hospital a person with an alcohol problem who has a history of one or more criminal offenses while under the influence of alcohol?

HYPOTHETICAL CASE EXAMPLE: T.A., a 40-year-old white, separated, Irish-Catholic male who is an officer in the military, was arrested early one Sunday morning when he went to his estranged wife's home after a wild drinking party and began throwing rocks at her windows, smashing them. When she came out in order to stop him, he struck her, breaking her nose and causing one of her front teeth to come loose. Her neighbor contacted the police and A's wife had him arrested.

The next day T.A.'s wife called a mental health professional at a local woman's center and asked three questions:

1. Would T.A. be held culpable for the crime of public intoxication?
2. Would T.A. be found legally responsible for the destruction of property and personal harm he caused her while under the influence of alcohol?
3. What role may the courts request psychiatry to play in A's disposition?

DISCUSSION

This hypothetical case raises three broad issues that will be discussed in the following order; the characterization of alcoholism as a disease, the chronic alcoholic's responsibility for criminal acts other than alcoholism and the role of psychiatry in the legal disposition of the alcoholic offender.

1) Is chronic alcoholism considered to be a disease by various courts; if so, what are the legal consequences of that characterization? The impetus behind the growing recognition by some courts that alcoholism, particularly chronic alcoholism, is a disease was the decision in the Robinson case in the early 1960s. This case, discussed in the previous chapter, was concerned with narcotics addiction, but the principles articulated were quickly applied to the legal understanding of chronic alcoholism. In effect the Robinson case, decided by the U.S. Supreme Court, held that it would be violating the protections of the Bill of Rights to penalize individuals simply for being drug addicts. It arrived at this decision through recognizing that narcotic addiction is a disease and that addicts are consequently sick individuals who should be treated rather than punished.

Two cases were decided in the mid-1960s by different U.S. Courts of Appeals that applied essentially the same reasoning behind the Robinson decision to chronic alcoholism. The first of these cases was the precedent-setting Driver case which was decided in 1966 by the Court of Appeals for the Fourth Circuit covering Virginia, West Virginia, North and South Carolina and Maryland (Driver vs. Hinnant, 1966). In this case the defendant was sentenced to be imprisoned for two years by a North Carolina court for the crime of public intoxication, having been convicted for the same offense over 200 times during his adult life of about 40 years; he had already spent most of his life incarcerated for chronic alcoholism. On this occasion the defendant pleaded that it was cruel and unusual punishment in violation of the Eighth Amendment to penalize him for chronic alcoholism which he argued was a disease effectively destroying the power of free will. His case was appealed through the various state courts until it reached the Federal Circuit Court of Appeals which upheld his argument.

The Fourth Circuit Court of Appeals in the Driver case argued that chronic alcoholism is fundamentally an involuntary act and therefore the chronic alcoholic can not be charged with a criminal act that requires the presence of criminal intention *(mens rea)*. The court stated that the defendant's chronic alcoholism was a condition that "has destroyed the power of his will to resist the constant, excessive consumption of alcohol; his appearance in public in that condition is not his volition, but a compulsion symptomatic of the disease; and to stigmatize him as a criminal for this act is cruel and unusual punishment." In the Easter case adjudicated later that year by the D.C. Circuit Court of Appeals, the decision of the Driver case was adopted for the District of Columbia (Easter vs District of Columbia, 1966). The U.S. Supreme Court in the Powell case in 1968 had an opportunity to substantiate the holdings of the Driver and Easter cases. However, it appeared to take a contrary position for it rejected the claim of the defendant Powell that his conviction for public drunkenness offended the Eighth Amendment. On close examination, however, the Supreme Court's holding was not incompatible with either the Driver or Easter cases in that it rejected Powell's claim because he was unable to establish the factual premises in his defense of involuntariness. If the defendant would have been able to present the necessary evidence to show that he was compelled to drink and that his appearance in public was

involuntary, the Supreme Court would have most likely arrived at the same conclusion as the earlier Driver and Easter cases.

As it now stands the decision in the Driver and Easter cases are binding in the
jurisdictions that are covered by those courts. Other parts of the country either
rely on the traditional criminal process to take care of alcoholics and allow them
to be penalized for public drunkenness, or they have instituted new therapeutic
measures such as requiring them to attend clinics or be hospitalized instead of
being imprisoned and fined. Interestingly, although the Powell decision did not
overrule those of the Driver and Easter cases because it did not get at the substantive issue of whether chronic alcoholism is a disease which affects the individual's
freedom of will, had it in fact upheld the argument of the defendant, all the
jurisdictions in the country would have had either to provide treatment for the
involuntary public drunk, or to permit him to remain free of criminal penalties.

An important distinction made by both the Driver and Easter cases is the one
between chronic alcoholism and excessive drinking. Both of these cases require a
person to be excused for the public intoxication he might suffer from chronic
alcoholism. If he were apprehended by the police for one or a few bouts of
excessive drinking he would not qualify for special treatment according to the
findings of these cases. Chronic alcoholism is associated with involuntary behavior
even though it might be argued that the first drink taken by the chronic alcoholic
required a conscious and voluntary decision on his part; after the first drink and
a history of continuing alcohol consumption the behavior becomes involuntary. On
the contrary, episodes of excessive drinking do not result in behavior which cannot
be controlled by the participant. It is very difficult on medical grounds alone often
to differentiate between those that consume alcohol and are chronic alcoholics and
those who have not lost their "free" will but nonetheless drink excessively. In
addition to this difficulty, it could be shown that by treating the excessive alcoholic
as one who possesses freedom of choice and is therefore legally accountable for his
conduct, the courts are actually creating an incentive for the consumer of alcohol
to move closer to the chronic condition when he would no longer be held culpable
for being in the illegal state of public intoxication. Persuasive as these arguments
are against distinguishing chronic alcoholism from other types of alcoholic behavior, the distinction has effectively been accomplished in both the Driver and
Easter cases and also in the discussions of the Supreme Court in its evaluation of
the Powell case.

Returning to the hypothetical case, it would be safe to conclude that the defendant would not qualify as a chronic alcoholic, at least not on the basis of the
information presented. The courts abiding by the Driver and Easter decisions
would view the defendant's conduct as resulting from one episode of excessive
drinking and therefore would not see him as acting without freedom of choice. If,
however, there had been additional information suggesting that the defendant
had a long history of frequent excessive drinking sprees and that he rarely had
periods when he was not to some extent under the influence of alcohol, the
distinction between excessive drinking and chronic alcoholism might be very
difficult for the court to prove, and they might choose to classify him as a chronic
alcoholic.

Before ending this section, it is important to note that the President's Commission on Law Enforcement and the Administration of Justice in their 1967 report
recommended that drunkenness should not be considered a crime and that public
health programs for treatment and rehabilitation should be substituted for the

traditional criminal system in handling these offenders. In response to that report and to a second presidential commission which evaluated crime in the District of Columbia and made similar recommendations, the District of Columbia passed the D.C. Alcoholic Rehabilitation Act. This act repealed its traditional law that viewed public intoxication as a criminal offense, except under those extreme circumstances where persons or property are endangered, and clearly states that public intoxication is a public health problem and that the chronic alcoholic is "a sick person who needs, is entitled to, and shall be provided appropriate medical, psychiatric, institutional, advisory, and rehabilitative treatment services . . . for his illness." Other jurisdictions have similarly shifted their positions.

2) Is the chronic alcoholic responsible for criminal acts committed while under the influence of alcohol? In the hypothetical case T.A. injured his estranged wife and destroyed some of her property. In the previous section the unlikelihood of his being considered a chronic alcoholic and thereby exempt from criminal prosecution was discussed. However, for the sake of argument, let us assume that the court classified him as a chronic alcoholic and refused to convict him on the charge of public drunkenness; would he still be culpable for these other criminal offenses? More than likely the answer would be in the affirmative. Neither the Driver or Easter cases recommended that the chronic alcoholic be exempt from all criminal charges; in fact the court in the Driver case explicitly stated that the chronic alcoholic would not be exempted from being judged for other criminal activities, "With respect to other behavior—not characteristic of confirmed chronic alcoholism—he would be judged as would any person not so afflicted." Even the President's Crime Commission recommended that although drunkenness should not in itself be considered a criminal offense, "disorderly and other criminal conduct accompanied by drunkenness should remain punishable as separate crimes."

Of course, the fact that alcoholism *per se* does not excuse one from criminal conduct does not mean that other remedies are not available for the drinker who while intoxicated commits a serious crime that has as one of its elements the requirement that specific intent be shown on the part of the offender. For example the fact that a murderer was drunk when he committed the crime would probably not exonerate him completely from the act, but might justifiably be used to reduce the offense from perhaps first-degree murder which requires a specific premeditated purpose to a lesser crime like murder in the second degree or even manslaughter. In some cases the fact that the offender was drunk when the crime occurred has resulted in acquittal, especially where the crime in question required the showing of criminal intention or *mens rea*. The psychotic drinker is likely to be excused completely from criminal guilt because he can reasonably employ the insanity defense. But the distinction between the psychotic drinker and the chronic alcoholic is often vague; in some states, particularly where the Durham or "product" rule is operative, alcoholism may be classified as a "mental disease or mental defect" and result in a successful insanity plea.

The most difficult problem for the courts has been in determining the link between the disease of alcoholism and the crime as well as establishing whether the alcoholic condition was sufficient to preclude freedom of choice. Surely no one would agree to a blanket rule that chronic alcoholism affects free will and therefore should be considered an excuse for all criminal activities. Medical knowledge has not yet reached a level of sophistication establishing when and under what conditions alcoholism does meet the criteria of eliminating voluntary behavior on the part of the consumer. At best the chronic alcoholic is placed in the position of any other person accused of criminal conduct, that is he must show that he lacked criminal intention *(mens rea)* or the voluntariness of his act *(actus reus)*. If he is successful in achieving an acquittal, perhaps because he established "criminal insanity" under the inclusive insanity defense, he may still be liable to a suit for damages, as discussed in the chapter on the insanity defense. A "mentally ill" patient is still liable for personal and property damages even though he is acquitted for the criminal act. In the event that the defendant in the hypothetical case is acquitted for criminal conduct, he can still be sued by his wife for damage to her windows and her person.

3) What role has psychiatry been given by the legislature and the courts in the disposition of chronic alcoholics? Nearly 30 states have procedures for the hospitalization and treatment of seriously disturbed chronic alcoholics. These involuntary commitment procedures are usually part of the laws dealing with commitment of the mentally ill. An alcoholic can be institutionalized through voluntary application or can be committed through medical certification or judicial order. The period of commitment is usually indeterminate based on when the alcoholic is considered cured.

Perhaps the most difficult feature of these commitment procedures is that they do not define the degree of alcoholism warranting civil confinement. Some state statutes attempt to deal with this feature by requiring that the alcoholic reach the stage of habitual use where he can no longer exert self-control over his drinking, or that his condition makes him potentially dangerous to himself or to others. Other states require that before he can be committed he has to have been convicted of public intoxication at least once.

Where the Driver or Easter case is operative the chronic alcoholic who is excused from the crime of public drunkenness is likely to be channeled into a therapeutic program. This might require that he be treated either as an outpatient or through hospitalization. Statutes such as the one passed in 1968 in the District of Columbia also provide for treatment of the chronic alcoholic. As a result of such court decisions and statutory changes, psychiatry has been given an expanded role in the disposition of the chronic alcoholic.

REFERENCES

Amsterdam A (1967): Federal constitutional restrictions on crimes of status, crimes of general obnoxiousness, crimes of displeasing police officers, and the like. Criminal Law Bull 3:205

Brakel SJ, Rock RS (1971): The Mentally Disabled and the Law (revised ed) Chicago, University of Chicago Press

District of Columbia Alcohol Rehabilitation Act, (1968) Pub L No 90–542, 82 Stat 618

Driver vs Hinnant, (1966) 356 F 2d 761 (4th Cir)

Easter vs District of Columbia, (1966) 124 US App DC 33, 361 F 2d 50 (en banc)

Greenawalt K (1969): Uncontrollable actions and the eighth amendment: Implication of Powell vs Texas. Colorado Law Rev 69:927

Hutt PB, Merrill RA (1969): Criminal responsibility and the right to treatment for intoxication and alcoholism. Georgetown Law J 57: 835

Kirbens SM (1968): Chronic alcohol addiction and criminal responsibility. Am Bar Assn J 54:877

Kittrie N (1971): The Right to be Different: Deviance and Enforced Therapy. Baltimore, Johns Hopkins Press

Powell vs Texas, (1968) 392 US 514

President's Commission on Crime in The District of Columbia Report (1966), pp. 474–503

President's Commission on Law Enforcement and Administration of Justice, Task Force Report (1967): Drunkenness. pp. 1–6

Robinson vs California, (1962) 370 US 660

Slaby AE, Tancredi LR (In Press): Collusion for Conformity, New York, Jason Aronson

Stern G (1969): Handling public drunkenness: Reforms despite Powell. Am Bar Assn J 55:656

Tao LS (1969): Psychiatry and the utility of the traditional criminal law approach to drunkenness offenses. Georgetown Law J 57:818

15 DIVORCE PROCEEDINGS

Today the process of obtaining a divorce is becoming much simpler for the average American. To bring into the open for review by the courts extremely personal information that may be psychologically damaging to spouse and children is no longer necessary, and some states, such as California, have gone so far as to implement a "no-fault" system for obtaining divorces. This change in attitude has had little impact thus far on divorce when one of the parties is mentally ill. In fact it has only been in the past several decades that divorce has been granted on the grounds of mental disability, and even under these conditions the mentally ill partner is considerably protected by the law. Although the argument is strong that a wife with several children would be better off separated from a mentally-ill husband, especially when frequent and prolonged hospitalizations interrupt their marriage and family life, under certain conditions the law will bend over backwards to defend the helpless member of society. The mentally-ill, hospitalized patient is considered helpless and the law consequently imposes major impediments in the way of actions against such patients, including divorce actions.

HYPOTHETICAL CASE EXAMPLE: D.P., a 36-year-old white, male, executive of a textile mill was hospitalized for a psychotic episode during which he had begun to spend large amounts of money and to frequent bars, often spending nights with prostitutes. This behavior was totally inconsistent with his former personality when he was reluctant to spend money and to socialize. His wife also noticed that he was becoming increasingly excitable, often speaking so rapidly that it was nearly impossible to follow his thoughts.

On the day of admission to the hospital he was hallucinating actively and showing suspiciousness, claiming that his family intended to harm him. Both of the daughters, ages 13 and 9, were in therapy at a child guidance center for recurrent attacks of overwhelming anxiety. Apparently the marriage had never been a happy one with both parties having a number of extramarital affairs. The issue of divorce had come up various times, most recently three weeks before he became sick and required hospitalization. On that occasion he had come home from work furious to learn that his wife was planning to visit her parents for a couple of weeks. In the course of the argument he became physically assaultive causing injuries to her arms that required medical attention. She had been reflecting over this latest abuse and had made up her mind that a separation and divorce were appropriate measures, when he became sick and was hospitalized.

Despite her husband's present condition, the wife was now convinced that a separation and divorce should be pursued. She asked her attorney if there were any likelihood of her being successful at this time in a divorce action.

DISCUSSION

Mental illness may be grounds for divorce according to the statutes of at least 30 states if it develops following marriage. When at the time of a marriage, mental disabilities such as epilepsy and mental deficiency exist a divorce cannot be granted and an annulment may be the only recourse available for dissolving the marriage. The interesting feature about the statutes that allow mental illness to be the grounds for divorce is that they allow a medical condition to be the basis for divorce. For the most part divorce is the accepted remedy when an injurious act against one spouse can be imputed to the other, such as physical or mental cruelty, adultery, child neglect or abuse, *et cetera.* Mental illness can hardly be interpreted as the responsibility or fault of the afflicted person; by allowing mental illness to be a basis for divorce, the law has made divorce possible without the requirement of establishing fault.

There are probably several reasons why the statutes of over 30 states make divorce possible on these grounds. There has been a gradual evolution in torts law as well as in domestic relations laws to minimize the role that "fault" should play in court decisions. To require a showing of injury in marriages in order to justify divorce is artificial since most often both parties harm each other in the marital relationship. The imputing of fault to one party is an inaccurate characterization of a marriage gone wrong. Even in the field of accident law when one might assume it would be relatively easy to describe what happens when two automobiles collide, "fault" has been difficult if not impossible to establish. Secondly, it increasingly seems unfair to force two people to stay married when one spouse is essentially insane. In certain circumstances when the disease is severe, a spouse can be deprived of the advantages of marriage, particularly companionship, for many years. And, third, a mentally-ill parent may be damaging to his child's psychological and social development; a child also may adopt some of the aberrant characteristics of the psychotic parent.

Even though divorce can be obtained because of mental illness, the terms of many of the statutes make it almost impossible. Except for Utah all of the states that have provisions for divorcing a mentally-ill spouse require that the mental condition persist over a period of time. Nearly half of the states specify that the mental condition last for at least five years, while others specify two or three years of mental disability. Most statutes, however, contain the provision that the condition be incurable, and more than half specify that medical testimony, often of more than one medical expert, must be given to establish that the mental illness is "incurable."

In most cases this provision effectively precludes the possibility of a divorce. Except for those organic diseases like the presenile dementias—Pick's or Alzheimer's disease, *et cetera*—or cases of insanity that result from traumatic head injury, it is nearly impossible to determine if a mental illness is incurable. This is particularly true since the major factor for determining incurability is whether the condition is responsive to acceptable treatment as determined by the length of time the patient spends in a mental institution. With the development of sophisticated antipsychotic medication, like chlorpromazine and related drugs, patients may be released from hospitals without achieving a full recovery from their disease. By the same token, patients may be kept in the hospital not because their condition is incurable but because staffing is inadequate to care for all the patients who could benefit from existing treatment. Using the length of time spent in a hospital, therefore, as a measure of curability is an undependable indicator. But perhaps even more important, few competent psychiatrists are willing to testify that nonorganic mental illnesses, like schizophrenia, manic–depressive illness, involutional melancholia and psychotic depression are incurable, yet these are the most common types of mental illness in the adult population.

Returning to the hypothetical case, it is unlikely that the wife would ever be able to bring a divorce action based on mental illness. Her husband has been mentally ill for a very short period of time and, furthermore, appears to suffer from a condition (probably manic–depressive illness) that would hardly be classified as "incurable" in the strict definition of that term. Manic–depressive illness is characterized by long periods of relatively normal functioning and may be effectively controlled with newer medications like lithium carbonate. However the wife in this case has another option available. She can claim that the divorce is justifiable on the basis of physical cruelty, evidenced before her husband became mentally ill.

Many courts when confronted with alternative grounds for divorce will allow the spouse's mental illness to be a defense against the divorce action. This would be the usual position if the injury had occurred while the spouse was mentally ill. The court applies a rule for determining responsibility similar to the one used in criminal cases where insanity is pleaded—a rule like the M'Naghten or ALI Test which require that the patient be able to differentiate right from wrong and possibly to show that he is able to conform his conduct to the requirements of the law. If in fact it can be shown that the spouse's mental condition did not prevent his understanding the nature of his act and that it was wrong, the divorce might be granted.

The wife in this case is claiming that her husband assaulted her physically before he became mentally ill. Under these circumstances his mental illness would not be a valid defense against divorce. The lawyer might claim that the patient's condition was in its early stages at the time he hit his wife, but it would be difficult with only the information presented here to convince the court that his mental condition had reached the point where he could no longer tell the difference between right and wrong; furthermore, the history of an incompatible marriage and frequent extramarital affairs would support the wife's case.

Now one might question whether the patient in this case could bring a divorce action. When illness has developed after marriage, mental patients are generally prevented from seeking a divorce. Because of delusions and bizarre thinking, mental patients frequently interpret the thoughts and actions of a spouse in a distorted manner. If divorce were encouraged among the mentally ill, many would likely regret such actions when they recovered. As a result only two states, Massachusetts and Alabama, permit mental patients to sue for divorce through the actions of a guardian or close friend.

In addition to the major issue of the effect that mental illness has on divorce proceedings, two related questions raised by the case of D.P. are of particular importance:

1) What is the role of the psychiatrist or mental health worker in divorce proceedings? Often the psychiatrist is called into court to evaluate various aspects of the issues presented in divorce proceedings involving mental patients. He may be asked to testify as to whether or not the spouse's mental condition could be cured. When mental illness is not the basis for a divorce action, the psychiatrist might be asked to establish whether the mentally-ill patient was capable of distinguishing right from wrong at the time an injury was committed and should be held responsible for his conduct. If the psychiatrist determines that the patient's condition prevented him from making this distinction a divorce might be prevented by the court.

There are the more delicate cases involving children, either in divorce actions or custody hearings. For example the healthy spouse claims that the mentally-ill husband beats one of his children so severely that on at least one occasion hospital treatment was required. The issue of child abuse might be used both to support the divorce action and to insure that the wife is given custody of the children. The court may request the child to testify that she was physically abused by her father. This could be a traumatic experience for a young girl, not only because she would have to testify against her father, but also because her testimony might serve as the basis for granting the divorce to the mother. By testifying she stands to lose her father and "family" and much guilt might ensue. If her father were being criminally prosecuted for child abuse, the daughter would be required to testify as would any adult who had been injured by another. In a civil case the psychiatrist might be successful in minimizing the trauma to the child either by disclosing the possible harmful effects of the child testifying to the mother, who might then elect to avoid using her child as the grounds for divorce, or by requesting that the proceeding be as informal as possible with little emphasis on the child's testimony.

With regard to the patient's psychiatrist he is obligated by virtue of the rule of "privileged" communication to disclose nothing under testimony unless the patient allows him to by waiving his rights of confidentiality. Of course there are situations when the privileged communication rule has little effect on the disclosure of psychiatric information. One such qualification to the rule in some states has been in custody hearings when a patient's therapist may be asked to reveal information about his patient which might be germane to the court's decision regarding who should have custody of the children. The psychiatrist may disclose information without fear of becoming involved in a suit for damages and breach of confidentiality.

2) Under what circumstances is an annulment a reasonable alternative to divorce when a mentally ill patient is involved? Before discussing the issue of annulment, it is important to emphasize the strong prohibitions against marriage, dis-

cussed in chapter 7, when one of the partners suffers from a mental disability. For the most part these prohibitions are based on three reasons: First, a mentally-ill person is unlikely to understand the nature of the marriage contract and therefore will be unable to consent to the agreement; second, certain kinds of mental illness, whether genetically or environmentally determined, seem to run in families and it would be to society's benefit to avoid such unions; and, third, mentally-ill persons tend to be unfit as parents despite the fact that their condition might be inherited. Unfortunately, despite the soundness of the arguments against such marriages, they do occur, partly because the prohibitions against them are nearly impossible to enforce. Except for the hospitalized patient who is under the strict regulations of an institutional structure, such sanctions against marriage have not been effective even though some states threaten criminal punishment of all parties involved including the clerk who issues the license. As a result many states, aware of the problems of enforcing sanctions against marriage, instead permit divorce or annulment as a reasonable relief to a marriage that involves a mentally-disabled person.

For a marriage to be valid the parties must have at least a reasonable understanding of the responsibilities incurred in the marriage relationship. This test of competency is not as severe as the level of competency required to transact business or form contracts. At least it is not so severe in most states, although at least eight states including New York require the same test of competency for marriage as for entering into other contractual relationships. Merely the presence of a delusion or hallucination or even mental retardation does not automatically nullify a marriage. The important ingredient in such a decision is whether or not there was the capacity to understand the marriage relationship at the time the event occurred. Therefore a schizophrenic patient would be considered validly married if the ceremony occurred during a lucid interval.

In most states mental incompetency is grounds for annulment. Some states explicitly hold that mental incompetency will void the marriage, which means in effect that the marriage never existed. This stipulation can have significant consequences in terms of property rights, for if the marriage never existed then the property accrued during the relationship would not be shared between the two parties. Furthermore, a marriage that can be void is subject to attack by a third person after the death of one of the parties, and could result in depriving the surviving spouse of inheritance and property rights. In addition children of a void union could be considered illegitimate. Most states that allow voiding, however, declare that children from these relationships are legitimate, but other features of a marriage like the sharing of property are often ignored when the marriage is called into question by one of the spouses or a third interested party. In order to favor the innocent party the trend has been in the direction of viewing marriages where one of the spouses does not meet the competency test as "voidable" (in contrast to "void") wherein the bond is valid until actually dissolved through a court determination. More and more states avoid any mention of voidability in their statutes, stating simply that mental incompetency at the time of the marriage is grounds for annulment. The law assumes that a person who enters a marriage was legally competent to do so; the burden of proof that mental incompetency was present at the time of the marriage lies with the party seeking the annulment.

REFERENCES

Allen RC, Ferster FZ, Weihofen H (1968): Mental Impairment and Legal Incompetency. New Jersey, Prentice Hall

Anthony R (1969): Clinical evaluation of children with psychotic parents. Am J Psychiatry 126:177

Brakel SJ, Rock RS (1971): The Mentally Ill and The Law (revised ed). Chicago, University of Chicago Press

Campbell vs Campbell, (1941) 242 Ala 141, 5 So 2d 401

Comment (1956): The mentally ill and the law of contracts. Temple Law Rev 29:380

Curran WJ, Shapiro ED (1970): Law, Medicine and Forensic Science. Boston, Little Brown

Davidson HA (195): Forensic Psychiatry. New York, Ronald Press

Deutsch A (1946): The Mentally Ill in America. New York, Columbia University Press

Green MD (1940): Public policies underlying the law of mental incompetency. Michigan Law Rev 38:1189

Guttmacher MS, Weihofen H (1952): Psychiatry and The Law. New York, WW Norton

Harper FV (1952): Problems of The Family. Indianapolis, Bobbs-Merrill

Libai D (1969) The protection of the child victim of a sexual offense in the criminal justice system. Wayne Law Rev 15:977

Massachusetts Annotated Laws (1955) 208, Section 7 (Supp 1968)

Robitscher JB (1966): Pursuit of Agreement: Psychiatry and The Law. Philadelphia, JB Lippincott

PART 4

THE **MENTAL HEALTH PROFESSIONAL** AS **DEFENDANT**

16 INADEQUATE CARE

The issues discussed here and in the next two chapters are broad and deal not so much with specific issues, but rather with the general responsibilities of a therapist or an institution when assuming the privilege of caring for a mentally-ill patient. When a psychiatric clinician elects to care for an individual, save in those circumstances where he assumes the role of a consultant and it is understood that the patient is being seen for a time-limited assessment of his mental condition, the clinician has a continuing responsibility to treat the patient until the patient recovers from his illness, until the patient formally informs the therapist that he no longer desires to continue in treatment or until the therapist informs the patient that he wishes to discontinue his services.

While there are certain circumstances which force a clinician to discontinue services, such as when the clinician moves to another city or develops an illness that precludes any professional activity, there are other situations when reasons for cessation of treatment may not be so apparent. In these situations the question of violation of the ongoing ethical responsibility to a patient is raised and the legal issue of *abandonment* emerges.

1. What happens if a psychiatric clinician abruptly discontinues his services without allowing the patient sufficient time to find a new therapist? The reasons for termination vary and may include instances when the clinician no longer has time because of other commitments, academic, clinical, or otherwise.

2. What happens if a clinician fails to respond to an emergency request from a patient? Obviously in psychiatry it is not always easy to define what is really an emergency as some patients' behaviors are characteristically manipulative and angry. In the latter case telephone calls outside a patient's regular appointments may not really represent true emergencies but rather a continuing pattern of a patient trying angrily to control his environment. This would

not be the case however with an individual who is acutely psychotic, homicidal or suicidal. In such instances, the clinician has an immediate responsibility to provide the needed service which may include hospitalization.

3. What if a psychiatric clinician goes on vacation without making arrangements for the care of his patients by an individual of comparable competence? Patients should know who the covering therapist is and that therapist should know who the patients are.

In addition to abandonment, the question of *inadequate care* may be raised when a patient is *promised* a cure for a particular ailment by a clinician but never gets well after a protracted course of expensive therapy. What constitutes a real promise as opposed to an optimistic prognosis may not be clear to some patients.

HYPOTHETICAL CASE EXAMPLE: I.C., a 55-year-old, white, divorced alcoholic called his therapist after skipping two appointments to tell him that he had been drinking more than usual and was extremely depressed. He had been fired two weeks previously from a job as a janitor he had held for eight months.

He told his therapist that he had difficulty falling asleep and had been waking at three o'clock in the morning for the previous ten days. His appetite had diminished considerably and he had lost 15 pounds in the past three weeks. He said he felt that he wanted to "end it all", much as he did following his divorce three years earlier when he attempted suicide by locking himself in the garage with the car's motor running. His son found him that time; following a brief hospitalization he began therapy with his current therapist. The clinician listened patiently but told I.A. he had to catch a plane in four hours for a vacation in Europe, and warned him not to do anything "crazy" until they had a chance to talk when he returned from his two-week vacation. He said, furthermore, that he would call a pharmacy to leave a prescription for some phenobarbital so that the patient would be able to sleep. The patient later picked up the phenobarbital tablets and successfully commited suicide by overdose the same night after calling his daughter to tell her what had happened that afternoon. At the funeral when I.A.'s daughter recounted that her father had told her that he had attempted to see his psychiatrist but was only given a prescription for "sleeping tablets", a friend told her to first check the truth of the story by going to the pharmacist and then consult a lawyer about suing for malpractice.

DISCUSSION

The area of medical malpractice is a complicated one with many facets, but our discussion here will be limited to a few of the basic principles of medical malpractice as they relate to the practice of psychiatry. First of all, medical malpractice refers to an act of negligence, incompetency or carelessness on the part of a psychiatrist or mental health worker that results in harm or damage to a patient. Implicit in the definition of medical malpractice is that the practitioner has done something wrong or has failed to render an appropriate medical service. This is not to say that a psychiatrist cannot make an honest mistake in diagnosis or in planning for treatment. After all, the practitioner is not guaranteeing a cure and when a patient is critically ill with obscure symptoms, mistakes can be made by the very best psychiatrists.

The standards that measure negligence or malpractice are based on the kind of care that is provided by most of the physicians in psychiatry in that community—a standard of care based on local practices. Negligence, therefore, would be the failure to exercise that level of care that most psychiatrists or mental health workers in the community provide. Whereas most jurisdictions maintain the locality rule, *i.e.*, those standards of the community, there is a growing trend toward developing national standards of care. The locality rule has been refuted in several recent court cases involving medical malpractice. The landmark case was decided in Massachusetts in 1968—the Belinkoff case—in which an anesthesiologist administered an excessive dose of a spinal anesthetic to a woman during delivery; several hours after the birth of her child the patient attempted to get out of bed, but her left leg was weak causing her to fall and injure herself (Brune vs. Belinkoff, 1968). A specialist from Boston which was over 50 miles from the community where the event occurred testified that the dosage of the spinal anesthetic was excessive. The trial court applied the locality rule, dismissing the statements by the "expert." The case, however, was appealed to the Supreme Court of Massachusetts which found that the level of care and skill representative of good medical practice is not limited to the community, but is rather the level of skill of most specialists, taking into consideration current medical advances and the available resources in the community (See also Christy vs Saliterman, 1970).

The test for negligence will be determined more and more on the standards of psychiatric care recognized nationally as the most effective in diagnosing and treating mental illness. Certainly if the results of recent court cases are any indication of a trend, the locality rule will no longer be the criterion for establishing acceptable conduct. In addition to court cases the emergence of Professional Standards Review Organizations (PSROs) should eventually result in national standards of care for each specialty. Medical care evaluation teams responding to the requirements of publicly financed programs like Medicare and Medicaid already are developing standards for treatment ranging from the number of visits appropriate for specific diseases to detailing the appropriate care for most of the illnesses a practitioner encounters. The PSROs will soon have their own network overseeing every specialty. When psychiatry becomes involved in the PSRO system, it too will be required to delineate treatment approaches and thereby define the limits of quality care.

Before examining some of the specific issues arising from the illustrative case, to discuss the way the expert witness is used in the court to establish malpractice is important. Usually the expert is presented with a hypothetical question based on the facts presented in the trial; he may be asked to give his opinion as to what a statement of facts might mean in terms of medical consequences. He is not allowed to draw inferences from the evidence or in any way attempt to judge the merits of the case. It is the prerogative of the jury not the expert to decide if the facts presented appear to be the truth. The hypothetical question presented to the expert assumes that the series of facts are true, and then asks what these facts might mean in terms of "cause" of illness, for example, or other medical issues. The information does not always have to be presented in a hypothetical form; if the testimony presented at the trial is uncontradicted an expert witness may be asked if he has formed an opinion from the testimony heard at the trial. For example, it might be established that an accident occurred during the administration of electroshock therapy (ECT) and the patient was injured. An expert might be asked if on the basis of the unrefuted accident, the injury could have developed. In addition to establishing the association between the event and subsequent injury, he could be asked to assist in defining the acceptable standard of care under these treatment conditions.

Returning to the illustrative case example, four broad issues are raised that will be discussed in the following order; psychiatric responsibility for abandonment of the patient, malpractice and the handling of the suicidal patient, injuries from various psychiatric procedures and the possibilities of a no-fault system for dealing with professional liability in psychiatry.

1) When does abandonment of the patient occur, and under what conditions would it be considered malpractice? The psychiatrist and mental health worker enter into a relationship with a patient essentially at their own discretion. They can elect not to establish a therapeutic relationship and be free of any possible legal consequences. However, once they do engage in a therapeutic encounter with a patient there is a duty and obligation to keep informed of the condition and administer to the needs of the patient during the period of his illness. The exception to this would be if there was a prior agreement that the time or scope of treatment would be limited.

Abandonment occurs when the therapist decides on his own to terminate his relationship with a patient when the patient still requires treatment. The therapist would not be held liable if the termination occurred with the consent of the patient or with sufficient notice so that the patient could obtain an appropriate substitute therapist. In addition, termination of treatment might be justified if the patient is totally uncooperative and refuses to accept the therapist's plan for treatment, or if in fact the condition of the patient is such that he no longer requires psychiatric attention. Where the patient elects to terminate treatment, it is important for the therapist carefully to record this decision so that he can not be held liable in the future for abandonment. When the therapist ends the relationship because he feels that the patient has recovered, he might be mistaken about the seriousness of the condition, in which case he makes the decision at his own risk and can be held liable for abandonment.

The fact that a therapist abandons a patient, whether intentionally or because of a mistaken notion about the patient's condition, is not in itself sufficient cause to establish negligence or malpractice. An injury must occur to the patient and it must be the result of the "abandonment." In other words, the court must find that had abandonment not occurred a satisfactory result would have been achieved. Therefore, the abandonment becomes both a necessary and sufficient cause of the injury suffered by the patient. In the hypothetical case the therapist's decision to go on vacation during a period of crisis for his patient was not in itself an abandonment. However, he failed to provide proper followup either by admitting the patient to a hospital or by arranging for another psychiatrist to care for this patient at a particularly critical period. Since the patient had attempted suicide in the past and now had all the signs of a major depression accompanied by suicidal ideation, the appropriate treatment would have been hospitalization.

2) What are the proper precautions to take in caring for a suicidal patient? In the hypothetical case the physician not only neglected to provide for adequate followup for this acutely ill patient, but significantly augmented the condition by prescribing phenobarbital, thereby providing the means for suicide. It is important in the treatment of a suicidal patient that he be carefully observed and that instruments that may be used for a successful suicide attempt are kept out of his reach. It is true that the most careful precautions do not necessarily prevent suicides from occurring, but by the same token, if an event is reasonably foresee-

able and controllable the psychiatrist must institute measures to prevent the injury or death. In the illustrative case the psychiatrist not only did not take reasonable precautions to prevent the suicide attempt, such as hospitalizing the patient, but he demonstrated very poor judgment by prescribing phenobarbital.

3) What are some other common psychiatric procedures which may cause injuries that could result in a malpractice action? There are three broad categories of psychiatric procedures which can result in legal problems primarily for psychiatrists. These procedures are involuntary commitment of patients, psychotherapy, and the use of mechanical or chemical therapies like electroshock treatment and insulin shock.

A. The issue of wrongful commitment. For the most part cases involving wrongful commitment have come out in favor of the psychiatrist. Courts have taken the position that a doctor–patient relationship does not develop when a psychiatrist examines a patient for possible commitment. In this role the psychiatrist is acting primarily under the directions of a state statute. Hence, even though he may make mistakes in his diagnosis of the patient, he has no special duty of care for which he could be held legally responsible. There are a few courts that have not accepted this position; instead they have held that the psychiatrist owes the patient the duty of making a mental examination with at least the usual care. Illustrative of this stance is the Kleber case which was decided in New York in 1963 [Kleber vs. Stevens, 1963]. In this case the patient alleged that the psychiatrist based his conclusions on her mental status on the statements made by her husband who was on bad terms with the wife at that time, rather than on the merits of a proper examination. The court concurred with the patient and held the psychiatrist liable. Of course, most courts would probably hold a psychiatrist liable if he committed a patient without performing a physical examination which is required by statute.

B. Malpractice and psychotherapy. It is very difficult to establish malpractice where verbal therapy is involved unless the psychiatrist or mental health worker has departed markedly from conventional treatment. The Hammer case was an example of a major departure from the usual treatment [Hammer vs. Rosen, 1960]. This case in 1960 was decided by the highest court of New York. The psychiatrist, Dr. Rosen, was accused of malpractice because he hit the patient during therapy. Dr. Rosen claimed that this was his method of therapy and that physical contact of this kind had been beneficial in a significant number of his patients. The New York court, however, felt differently even though several colleagues extolled the approach, and found the psychiatrist liable for malpractice in conducting improper treatment.

In addition to unusual therapy which allegedly damages the patient, courts have viewed cautiously social involvement of therapists and patients. One such case, the Landau case, occurred in England in the early 1960s; the patient fell in love with the psychiatrist and instead of terminating the treatment the psychiatrist engaged in social visits and outings with her [Landau vs. Werner, 1961]. According to the testimony the therapist did not make any improper advances, but the patient failed to recover and in fact actually got worse and attempted suicide. The court concluded that the therapist established such a strong transference relationship with the patient that it served to the detriment of her care.

C. The use of electroshock and similar therapies. Electroshock and insulin shock therapies are known to have a significant risk of complications. In the case of electroshock, which is by far the most commonly used shock therapy, it is expected that a relatively small percentage of cases will suffer from convulsions which may cause fractures of the bones and spine. Courts for the most part have been concerned with whether or not the patient was fully informed of the risks inherent in electroshock therapy. When it could be established that the patient was misled, as in the Woods case, the court would usually decide in favor of the patient [Woods vs. Brumlop, 1962]. The exceptions to the rule of full disclosure of the risks as discussed by the court in the Woods case should be limited to emergencies or situations where full discussion might alarm the patient.

Recent advances in the administration of electroshock have virtually ended the likelihood of secondary fractures and other injuries. The use of sedative and paralyzing agents minimize both convulsions and muscular contractions. Medical malpractice in the future will probably focus on the question of whether these medications were administered. If not, the therapist will be rightfully accused of not exercising due care in the treatment of his patient. In the case of insulin shock, informing the patient of the risks involved, such as convulsions and fractures, as well as the risk of potential brain damage from uncontrolled coma, is still critical in avoiding a successful malpractice suit.

4) Is it possible to design a no-fault system for handling untoward outcomes from psychiatric diagnosis and treatment? The current fault system for medical malpractice is characterized by many negative and few positive features. The fault system is a very costly system, much of the money going into legal and administrative fees; furthermore, to establish malpractice is difficult despite the fact that patients are often injured, perhaps unnecessarily, during therapy. When a patient wins, however, he may receive a very high settlement that in many ways does not reflect the injury sustained, but rather the capriciousness of the jury which is persuaded by "suffering" patients and the complaint of "pain" which is a nebulous, subjective experience. Also, the public trial has the added disadvantage of stigmatizing the physician whether he wins or loses the case. From a social justice standpoint the most serious failing of the fault system is that it does not compensate all those injured by medical intervention where such injuries could have been avoided.

One scheme that has been proposed to circumvent some of the inefficient features of the fault system is a medical adversity insurance system. The various medical specialities, including psychiatry, would be asked to define and identify their diagnostic and treatment injuries to the patient which have a relatively high degree of avoidability. If an untoward psychiatric event—for example, fractures from ECT—could be avoided by proper prevention or treatment, the patient should be compensated for the injury through the medical adversity insurance. The insurance would limit its payment to medical expenses resulting from the injury and loss of wages during the recuperative phase. Such a policy would be paid for by the provider—the physician or hospital—creating an incentive for them to be as careful as they can. This scheme has been worked out with some care for orthopedic surgery and anesthesiology; to begin to define events in psychiatry that all would agree are virtually avoidable given proper attention early should be possible. Some acts, like abandonment or neglecting to obtain informed consent for a psychiatric procedure, should possibly remain within the province of the court as they are tied to societal notions of professional conduct and therefore would be inappropriate in a no-fault system.

REFERENCES

Barnes vs Bovenmyer, (1963) 122 N.W. 2d 312 (Ia)

"The Best of Law and Medicine" (1968): Chicago, American Medical Association

Brune vs Belinkoff, (1968) 354 Mass 102, 235 NE 2d 793

Christy vs Saliterman, (1970) 288 Minn 144, 179 NW 2d 288 (This case is particularly relevant to psychiatry as the court allowed that a psychiatrist trained in Massachusetts and New Hampshire could testify on "national standards" in Minnesota.)

Collins vs State, (1965) 23 App Div 2d 898, 258 NYS 2d 238 (3rd Dept)

Curran WJ, Shapiro ED (1970): Law, Medicine and Forensic Science. Boston, Little Brown

Dawidoff DJ (1966): The malpractice of psychiatrists. Duke Law Journal 696.

Dawidoff DJ (1973): The Malpractice of Psychiatrists. Illinois, Charles C Thomas

Davidson HA (1965): Forensic Psychiatry. New York, Ronald Press

Hammer vs Rosen, (1960) 7 NY 2d 376, 165 NE 2d 756, 198 NYS 2d 65

Havighurst CC, Tancredi LR (1973): Medical adversity insurance—a no-fault approach to medical malpractice and quality assurance. Health and Soc 51:125

Woods vs Brumlop, (1962) 71 NM 211, 377 P 2d 520

Hirsh vs State, (1960) 8 NY 2d 125, 168 NE 2d 372

Kleber vs Stevens, (1963) 39 Misc 2d 712, 241 NYS 2d 497 (Sup Ct) Aff'd 20 App. Div 2d 896, 249 NYS. 2d 668 (1964)

Landau D (1967): Medical malpractice: Overturning locality rule used in determining a physician's standard of skill and care. Boston University Law Rev 48:710

Landau vs Werner, (1961) (Queens Bench) in Dawidoff DJ (1973): The Malpractice of Psychiatrists, Illinois, Charles C Thomas, p. 38

McCoid AH (1959): The care required of medical practitioners. Vanderbilt Law Review 12:549

Morse HM (1967): Psychiatric responsibility and tort liability. Journal of Forensic Sciences 12:305

Morse HN (1967): The tort liability of psychiatrists. Baylor Law Review 19:208

Perr R (1965): Liability of hospital and psychiatrist in suicide. Am J Psychiatry 122: 631

Tancredi L (1974): Identifying avoidable adverse events in medicine. Medical Care 12:935

Tancredi L, Woods J (1973): The social control of medical practice, Economic Aspects of Health Care. Edited by J McKinlay. New York, Prodist

17 INAPPROPRIATE CARE

Inappropriate care entails the use of techniques that have not been demonstrated to be helpful in a particular psychiatric condition and, furthermore, in some cases may be actually destructive. The tremendous range of theoretical orientations on the contemporary American psychiatric scene makes this not always a clear situation. Some psychologically oriented psychotherapists may be unequivocally convinced that psychoanalysis is the treatment of choice for a particular neurosis. Other therapists of a behaviorist bent may feel a conditioning approach is more appropriate for the same condition and an organic therapist may feel that medication is the best treatment. These issues are not easily resolved even at lengthy seminars called to arrive at a some homogeneous approach, (if that is desirable). One may be assured that if experts in the field of mental health disagree among themselves as to the best approach to a problem or recognize there may be several equally effective modes of treatment, a clinician who advocates one approach as opposed to another will not be found to use an "inappropriate" mode of treatment. There remain, however, some approaches that are so contrary to good clinical judgment that peer consensus would be that the method is inappropriate and perhaps in some cases contraindicated because of possible damage to a patient's well being.

HYPOTHETICAL CASE EXAMPLE: An eight-year-old child was brought to a psychiatrist by his parents because he was "uncontrollable." He frequently lied to them and stole from other students at school. He once had started a fire in his parents' bedroom but his father rapidly extinguished it. Both parents had periodically seen psychiatrists for recurrent marital problems and alcohol abuse. The psychiatrist felt that lysergic acid diethylamide should be given to the child. His rationale for its use was not entirely clear to the parents but supposedly it was to scare the child into altering his behavior. The parents signed a consent for the treatment and the child was given the hallucinogen. It induced in the child a psychosis which did not remit despite the administration of a phenothiazine medication. The child had recurring hallucinatory experiences several months later. The parents, horrified, called a physician friend who suggested they sue the therapist.

DISCUSSION

The psychiatrist in the hypothetical case resorted to the use of LSD, a drug not only of questionable value in the treatment of psychological conditions but one suspected of having serious consequences for the patient—especially the potentiality of inducing a major psychotic reaction. Controversy continues about the use of LSD in small doses to relieve the pain of chronic debilitating diseases (widespread malignancies, for example) and to cause a euphoric feeling in the terminally ill patient. Some consider the benefits to far outweigh the harm in this population. Because of the unfavorable recent publicity about LSD, it is rarely used even for this highly limited purpose.

The fact that the psychiatrist obtained the consent of the child's parents before giving the LSD is a powerful safeguard for the therapist against a malpractice suit. The psychiatrist or therapist must have the free and informed consent of a patient or guardian if he desires to use a new therapy; but, in addition, other conditions must be met to avoid a malpractice suit. First, there must be at least a reasonable chance that the new procedure will produce better results than existing therapies. Second, the hazards to the patient should not outweigh the benefits of the procedure. Experiments on appropriate laboratory animals or some experience with other patients is essential to predict accurately the benefits and risks of a new procedure.

There are circumstances when the courts may be inclined to disallow the above conditions. For example, when informed consent has been obtained and the patient is not seriously ill, treatments not expected to benefit the patient more than accepted therapies may be used if the risks to the patient are slight and the information which would be obtained would be significant to the society ar large. For example, it might be accepted knowledge that the appropriate treatment for chronic alcoholism does not include the use of drugs used for the treatment of psychosis—thorazine and lithium carbonate. By the same token, medicating alcoholic patients with lithium carbonate might be condoned because the risks are minimal and there is the chance that some will respond to the drug because of an underlying mood disorder. The likelihood of this occurring may be small, but the risks are minimal and the information obtained for the public benefit could be of major importance. Or when the patient is in a desperate condition, or on the verge of death, a physician may administer a drug or procedure even though it carries with it a high likelihood of serious side effects or even death, if the patient gives his informed consent and the dangers from the procedure are less than those of the patient's physical or mental disease. Hence, the use of LSD for the treatment of patients in the terminal and painful stages of a long-term illness may be justified.

In the hypothetical case the psychiatrist is placed in a particularly awkward position. There have been no studies to demonstrate that LSD is at all indicated even from an experimental–therapeutic standpoint, and evidence does exist showing that it can have serious side-effects. The use of minimal physical force as an adjunct to psychotherapy was condemned by the courts despite the support of some key figures in American psychiatry (Hammer vs. Rosen, 1960) as discussed in chapter 16. Were the psychiatrist brought to court there would be little or no support for his decision to use LSD. The range of acceptable psychotherapeutic techniques is wide in a psychotherapy case and the risks of serious harm were small, yet the court ruled against Dr. Rosen's unconventional approach to the patient.

The psychiatrist might claim that he gave the LSD as part of an experiment and that the patient and his family were aware of this. That a treatment is presented as experimental does not relieve the therapist of responsibility for injuries which might develop. The courts generally hold that a therapist who departs from the standard practices of similar specialists in his community does so at his own legal risk. The consent form signed by the patient's parents, even if it stated clearly that the treatment was experimental and if it carefully described the risks involved, would be of doubtful protection. The psychiatrist might not be held liable for having performed an unauthorized procedure having obtained consent, but the court would likely find that he was negligent in carrying out the therapy, especially if he did not adequately pretest its effects in laboratory animals or other patients. The psychiatrist might have a stronger case if he could show that other psychiatrists concurred with the advisability of the experiment.

If the psychiatrist is brought to court for medicating with LSD, he would probably be sued for a tort or wrongdoing in a civil procedure. The injured party may claim that the psychiatrist did not obtain informed consent and therefore performed an unauthorized procedure, or he may claim instead that the treatment was negligently conducted and that he suffered as a result. If the psychiatrist is held civilly liable he is expected to pay for the damages resulting from his inappropriate treatment. He may also be vulnerable to criminal prosecution if the procedure was dangerous and could be viewed as irresponsible. For the most part general offenses, criminal assault, homicide or mayhem, require proof of intent to injure another person on the part of the psychiatrist; however, the psychiatrist could also be held criminally responsible if the negligence were so gross as to amount to reckless disregard of the rights and safety of another person. Because of the medical reservations about LSD, the use of this medication for a mentally disturbed patient may well be interpreted as reckless disregard of his safety or gross negligence.

It is important to add to civil and criminal liability the fact that the psychiatrist may have also violated the standards of professional conduct and consequently his license to practice may be denied, suspended or revoked. The grounds for revocation or suspension of a license are defined by state statute and are usually characterized in vague terms such as unprofessional conduct, gross immorality or fraud. The state licensing agency is generally authorized to decide if licenses in medical practice should be revoked or suspended. The courts, however, may be called upon to enforce a revocation and some have suggested that licensing agencies should not assume the function of overviewing the activities of psychiatrists who engage in clinical investigation. Others feel that such agencies policing the conduct of all practitioners is appropriate.

Except for those cases where criminal prosecution is being considered, the major reason for a suit by an injured party is for the purpose of obtaining compensation for any injuries he has received. The expenses to a patient harmed during a psychiatric experiment can be quite significant. In addition to his medical expenses, the injured patient may also lose wages during the period of disability. As a result it has been proposed that one way to avoid the expenses—mostly legal—of a malpractice suit would be to provide a system of compensation for those injured in legitimate experiments. The system for compensation would be automatic so that patients injured in the course of a psychiatric experiment would be compensated to the extent of payment for additional medical services if needed, and for loss of wages during the time the patient is disabled. Such a system of compensation would essentially be a no-fault system; there would be no requirement to establish negligence on the part of the psychiatrist. The theoretical possibilities for this insurance compensation system have been worked out and would require (as with the no-fault system of medical malpractice discussed in Chapter 16) a fairly broad categorization of untoward outcomes that should be compensable. On the more practical level, a no-fault system for coverage of patients injured in medical and psychiatric research has been put into operation at the University of Washington to cover all research projects of a scientific nature involving humans. It is too soon to determine the effectiveness of this system of handling experimental injuries. Since the legal and administrative costs of a lengthy court proceeding are avoided and more people are likely to receive some compensation for their injuries—only a few actually win in a malpractice suit—the no-fault system should prove far more efficient than the existing system.

The following two questions are of special relevance to the overall topic of experimentation with psychiatric therapies.

1) What are the ethical issues surrounding experimentation with psychiatric therapies; should clinical experimentation have a major role in the care of the mentally ill? The issue of experimentation in mental health has recently become controversial. The introduction of new and effective therapies like behavior modification and psychosurgery are frightening to many because they have the potentialities of significantly altering the patient's personality. In the case of behavior modification the change in personality is directed at satisfying the desires of others, that is, the treatment may lead to behavior on the part of the patient which satisfies his family, community or even the society at large. Similarly, psychosurgery has the same potentiality of essentially inducing conformity in behavior and decreasing the individual's assertiveness. Electroshock and medication may have the same results, but they don't seem to create the public reaction that behavior control and psychosurgery do. In addition there have been some cases recently that directly affect the use of psychosurgery and behavior modification. There was a recent case in Michigan (Kaimowitz vs. Department of Mental Health of Michigan, 1973) when a court stopped the expenditure of state funds for use in an experimental psychosurgery program. Cases involving prisoners and others in vulnerable positions have successfully challenged the use of both psychosurgery and behavior modification by arguing that the patient has the right to refuse treatment.

By the same token, experimentation is essential in all facets of medicine; to understand if a certain diagnostic or therapeutic measure effectively serves the purposes for which it was developed and actually alters the natural course of a disease process, some form of experimentation is required. The limited resources of a society for supporting medical care demand that the system for providing care be not only effective but maximally efficient, and this can only be achieved if experimentation is conducted. At the same time that ethical and legal concerns have arisen about medical and psychiatric experimentation, there is the growing realization that it is ethically appropriate continually to test old and new diagnostic and therapeutic methods. As Cochrane (1971) clearly points out in his classic work, *Effectiveness and Efficiency—Random Reflections on Health Services,* the random clinical trial (RCT), a device used to compare two groups of patients by grouping them according to a method such as random numbers which is essentially independent from human choice has proved to be the most effective technique available for determining to what extent the outcomes of various treatment and diagnostic techniques are beneficial.

The value of the random clinical trial cannot be emphasized enough, especially for examining the effectiveness of existing diagnostic and therapeutic procedures. Such long held notions as the importance of coronary care units for the patient with an acute heart condition, and oral diabetic agents for the treatment of maturity-onset diabetes have been called into question by well controlled trials. Psychiatry likewise has a responsibility to evaluate its methods for diagnosis and treatment. It is a fundamental duty of all the therapeutic professions to reflect and test the accuracy of their scientific concepts.

Inevitably, however, a conflict is created. On the one hand there is the desire to test thoroughly the value of treatments, and on the other the obligation to provide the best possible care for the patient. Both sides of the conflict have their ethical justifications. The need for well controlled experiments, especially the use of the random clinical trial, has already been argued. To a great extent the obligations to the patient are served by informing him of the nature and risks of an experiment. But, in addition, there must be a reasonable likelihood that the benefits expected from the experimental therapy exceed the risks or disadvantages; and that in any case, the experimental procedure should benefit the patient as much or more than existing therapeutic measures. The most important protective requirement for the patient is that the procedure has been adequately pretested —most often through well-designed animal studies—before being used on the patient population.

2) In addition to informed consent what other devices are being considered to protect the subject of a clinical experiment or the patient requiring therapy? Informed consent has been considered the most important protective measure for the patient who participates in clinical research or who requires medical treatment. When the patient can demonstrate that he was not informed of the hazards of a psychiatric treatment, nor gave his consent, the psychiatrist has been held liable for a malfeasance. In the Mitchell case, for example, the psychiatrist failed to inform the patient of the risks associated with insulin shock and the patient suffered fractures of his vertebrae. The court found the psychiatrist liable for malpractice because he neglected to inform the patient of this possible side effect. Recent cases in the area of informed consent actually impose a duty on the therapist to inform the patient of risks associated with procedures even if he does not request such information.

But there are difficulties with "informed consent", especially where some information has been given to the patient but perhaps not enough to inform him fully of risks. It has often been very difficult to establish which risks the patient was aware of before he consented to the treatment program. Furthermore, it has been equally difficult to determine if the patient was of sufficient mental capacity to comprehend the information provided him. As a result various groups, in particular the National Institutes of Health (NIH), have been carefully evaluating other ways of regulating research involving patients. The major recommendations proposed so far are for setting up committees, such as consent or protection committees, ethical review boards and perhaps even a national body to set broad standards for experimentation.

The concept of the "consent" committee emerged from recent deliberations of the NIH committee on the Protection of Human Subjects. The reason for such committees in institutions receiving government support is to protect vulnerable groups who are often unable to exert free choice, such as prisoners, the mentally retarded and mentally ill, both adult and children. As the concept is now designed, the consent committee would serve an overview role, evaluating experimental projects before they are conducted to establish whether in fact they should be allowed. Such committees could prove quite useful in eliminating grossly unethical studies from being conducted in a health care setting. However, they may tend seriously to impede important scientific research or even prevent it from being completed where the ethical conflicts may be quite minor. There will be a tendency to delay approval of research projects that can be important in the mental health field. In addition such committees will be inclined to promote conservative research over research which, though more innovative, may in fact involve fewer risks. Equally important as these criticisms is that layers of committees simply mean more bureaucratic involvement in the therapeutic process which can be costly to society as well as expanding the administrative duties of therapists. More effective in the long run than additional committees which can stifle scientific progress would be a tightening of the legal standards for meaningful informed consent and the establishment of a compensation system for those injured—a no-fault system whereby the patient would be automatically compensated for medical expenses and loss of wages through a medical adversity insurance system.

REFERENCES

Beecher HK (1966): Ethics and clinical research. N Engl J Med 274:1354

Beecher HK (1959): Experimentation in man. JAMA 169:461

Beecher HK (1970): Research and The Individual Human Studies. Boston, Little Brown

Cobbs vs Grant, (1972) 104 Cal Rptr 505

Cochrane AL (1971): Effectiveness and Efficiency-Random Reflections on Health Services. London, The Nuffield Provincial Hospitals Trust

Davidson H (1965): Forensic Psychiatry. New York, Ronald Press

De Lange SA (1973): Ethical implications of psychosurgery. Psychiatr Neurol Neurochir 76:383

Halleck S (1974): Legal and ethical aspects of behavior control. Am J Psychiatry 131:381

Hammer vs Rosen, (1960) 7 NY 2d 376, 165 NE 2d 756, 198 NYS 2d 65

Havighurst CC, Tancredi LR (1973): Medical adversity insurance—a no-fault approach to medical malpractice and quality assurance. The Milbank Memorial Fund Quarterly: Health and Soc 51:125

Kaimowitz vs Department of Mental Health for the State of Michigan, (1973) 2 Prison Law Reporter

Katz J (1972): Experimentation with Human Beings. New York, Russell Sage Foundation

Mather HG, Pearson WG, Read KLQ, et al (1971): Acute myocardial infarction: Home and hospital treatment. Br Med J 7:334

McCoid AH (1957): A reappraisal of liability for unauthorized medical treatment. Minnesota Law Rev 41: 381

Mitchell vs Robinson, (1960) 334 SW 2d 11 (Mo) aff'd 360 SW 2d 673 (Mo 1962).

Myers MJ (1967): Informed consent in medical malpractice. California Law Rev 55:396

Note (1970): Restructuring informed consent: Legal therapy for the doctor-patient relationship. Yale Law J 79:1532

Plante ML (1968): An analysis of 'informed consent'. Fordham Law Rev 36:639

"Protection of human subjects, proposed policy" (1973). Federal Register 38:27882

Secretary's Commission on Medical Malpractice (1973): Report of The Secretary's Commission on Medical Malpractice. Washington, DC, Department of Health, Education and Welfare, US Government Printing Office

Tancredi L (In Press): The ethics quagmire and random clinical trials. Inquiry

18 INSTITUTIONAL LIABILITY

With the increasing use of nonphysician mental health professionals, the question of their responsibilities becomes an important issue. Not all these responsibilities are clearly defined; therefore, it is good practice for a psychiatric clinician who is not a physician to consult with a lawyer in regard to his legal responsibilities toward his patients in his state. To avoid violation of laws on medical licensure is a legal obligation. The burgeoning mental health field has in the past decade brought to the fore a number of unique issues; for instance, when a physician refers a psychiatric patient to a nonphysician therapist who accepts the patient into his care, is the doctor–patient relationship terminated as it would be if the referral were to another physician?

When a nonphysician clinician works for or under the direction of a physician, he is said to be the physician's "agent" and the physician is held responsible for the clinician's work. If he works for an institution, the institution may be liable. The patient injured by the nonmedical therapist may sue the physician under the doctrine of *respondeat superior* ("let the master respond"). This doctrine in effect allows the injured party to bring an action against the employer or in this case the physician because it is assumed that the employee is acting under the supervision of the superior. A psychiatrist may have several mental health workers assisting him in his practice but he must be aware of the fact that he can be held liable for the negligent act of any one of these therapists. Also, if the psychiatrist agrees to assist a nonmedical therapist in treating the patient with medication he is likewise potentially liable certainly for injuries that can be related to improper medication. Similarly, if the mental health worker works for an institution, the institution may be held liable.

HYPOTHETICAL CASE ILLUSTRATION: Late one Saturday evening, I.L., a 45-year-old white, Jewish widow of a well-known lawyer, was brought to the emergency room of a small community hospital by her married daughter. The receptionist called the house officer, an intern, to see the patient. The intern learned that the patient had not been feeling well. She had lacked much appetite since her husband's death three months previously, had lost about forty pounds and felt her insides were sawdust. Wringing her hands, she paced the floor continually and spoke of the guilt she had for not having loved her husband enough to keep him alive. Even though he had died of a malignant brain tumor, she felt she caused it. She stated she heard his voice each night begging her to come to join him. She was restless, sleeping only two to three hours a night. She seldom fell asleep before two o'clock in the morning and would usually be up at five. She was constipated and her mouth always seemed dry. Three years earlier, when her daughter left home to marry, the patient had attempted to kill herself by an overdose of barbiturates and alcohol. She was found unconscious by her husband at that time and brought to the hospital where she received intensive treatment for three days. She then had psychiatric care for a year doing quite well on a course of antidepressant medication and supportive psychotherapy. When the intern asked her if she had suicidal thoughts, she quite vehemently denied having any.

The intern carefully wrote down all the relevant features of the history and then decided that he could handle the matter himself, and that there was no need to consult a psychiatrist. In any case psychiatric consultation was not easy to obtain in the hospital. The intern gave the patient an appointment to come back in one week for an intake evaluation in the outpatient psychiatric clinic of the hospital.

Early the next morning, the patient, overdosed with barbiturates, was found in a comatose state by a neighbor who summoned an ambulance. After three days of treatment in an intensive care unit she was essentially recovered and was transferred to a medical unit for further care and psychiatric evaluation. The patient's son-in-law stated that they should sue the hospital because an intern had seen the patient and knowing her psychiatric history had failed either to admit her or to seek psychiatric consultation.

DISCUSSION

Until the early 1940s most community hospitals were essentially exempt from malpractice suits. There were several court cases then that held hospitals liable for negligence and some states began to change their legislation to allow hospitals to be sued like any other corporations for not meeting high standards of care. Under the notion of *corporate negligence* hospitals are responsible for a variety of administrative functions, selecting competent personnel and training them properly, assuring adequate supervision of employees and maintaining its equipment and buildings in an appropriate manner. Both profit and nonprofit hospitals have been usually considered liable for these corporate functions.

With regard to *vicarious liability*, the legal responsibility for the negligent acts of its individual employees (nurses, physicians, *et cetera*), certain institutions that meet the criteria defined by law that would make them charitable or nonprofit hospitals enjoy special status under a legal theory called "charitable immunity." This means that nonprofit hospitals can be held liable only for not using care in the selection of its employees, but not liable for injuries to patients that might be due to an employee's negligence. Recently, however, the doctrine of "charitable immunity" has been eroded by the courts in many states, so that in at least 28 jurisdictions total liability for negligence is imposed on hospitals whether profit or nonprofit.

There has even been a significant expansion of the duties that are considered part of the corporate responsibility of hospitals. A distinction used to be drawn between administrative and medical functions; hospital liability, except for negligent acts of its employees under the theory of vicarious liability (which has also undergone much expansion in recent years), had been limited to administrative negligence for it had been felt that corporations (hospitals) could not practice medicine in the traditional sense. But this distinction with regard to corporate responsibility has also broken down, particularly as a result of a landmark case decided in 1965—the *Darling* case (Darling vs. Charlestown Memorial Hospital, 1965).

In the Darling case the Illinois Supreme Court held a hospital liable for violating medical duties it owed to a patient. An 18-year-old male was treated for a fractured leg by a general practitioner at the emergency ward of a community hospital. The practitioner applied traction and placed the leg in a cast. Several days later the patient returned complaining of severe pain and the odor of decayed tissue was present. Unfortunately, the patient did not receive attention soon enough and it was necessary to amputate the leg. The patient and his family sued the hospital, and despite the fact that the general practitioner was not employed by the hospital, the court found the hospital negligent for allowing an unqualified doctor to perform orthopedic surgery and for not requiring consultation or review of treatment by a specialist. This decision redefined the role of the hospital in the practice of medicine. The court was not recommending that the hospital must actually control the medical practice of the physician, but rather that the standards of patient care are the joint responsibility of the physician and institution. Thus, the old notion that a corporation or hospital cannot practice medicine was refuted. Other cases following the Darling decision have even found an institution liable if it knew or should have known that a physician departed from acceptable standards of care (Fiorentino vs. Wenger, 1966).

Hospitals can be held liable for the negligent acts of their professional employees under the legal theory of vicarious liability, otherwise known as *respondeat superior*—the position that the employer is liable for the negligent act of employees, is often referred to as the "captain-of-the-ship" doctrine. This concept has recently been expanded in scope resulting in a shift away from the view of the physician as the "captain-of-the-ship" and, therefore, responsible for the negligent acts of hospital employees to the principle of holding the hospital or health care institution liable for such negligences (French vs Fisher, 1962; Kapuschinsky vs United States, 1966; Tonsic vs Wagner, 1974).

The latter doctrine of vicarious liability is particularly relevant to the hypothetical case. The intern is an employee of the hospital and consequently the hospital could be held liable for his negligent acts. In this illustration there would be a very strong case against the intern. There were many features of the patient's history and presentation to the emergency ward that suggested she was a high suicidal risk; information like the fact that she was a recent widow, had recently lost 40 pounds, had a previous history of a serious suicidal attempt and presented with symptoms of depression and suicidal ideation (such as hearing voices in the night), having a psychotic delusion about feeling like "sawdust," pacing the floors and being unable to sleep would indicate that she required at the very least hospitalization with suicide precautions.

By discharging the patient with the history and symptoms she presented, the intern was negligent. Of course he could be sued for his lack of appropriate care in his treatment of the patient. But more important from the standpoint of a suit and receiving a high award by the court, the hospital could also be sued, and the family would probably be quite successful in a malpractice action against both the intern and the hospital. If the physician covering the emergency room had not been an intern or an employee of the hospital but a general practitioner contracting his services to the hospital, the hospital might be liable under the theory of corporate negligence, especially if the jurisdiction followed the holding of the *Darling* case, or a similar holding. In such a situation one could argue that the hospital should be liable for allowing an unqualified physician to engage in sophisticated psychiatric diagnosis and treatment without consultation with a psychiatrist.

The important issue of this discussion is that the hospital or health care institution is becoming increasingly liable both for the acts of its employees and the medical care that it provides. The implication behind this trend is that the hospital acts as the primary provider of care, and as a result should be held legally responsible. Not all states have expanded the scope of legal notions like vicarious liability or corporate negligence, but there is definitely a move in that direction which will intensify with the advent of group practice and Health Maintenance Organizations (HMOs) on a large scale, as well as a national health insurance system that will probably result in the setting of high standards for the institutional providers of medical care.

In addition to the major considerations of institutional liability for the practice of medicine and psychiatry, this hypothetical case raises the problem of hospital responsibility for suicide and the broader issue of alternative approaches to compensating the patient who is injured in the hospital.

1) Can a hospital be held liable for suicide? Hospitals as well as psychiatrists have been held liable for a patient's death or injury shown to be due to the failure adequately to restrain or to control a patient under their care. Hospitals are more susceptible to malpractice suits than doctors because allegedly the inadequate care was a lack of appropriate watchfulness or control over the patient while in the hospital. This is the responsibility of the hospital and not the doctor. The doctor would be liable for a suicide if the care he provided were not reasonable, as in the illustrative case in Chapter 16 where the therapist prescribed phenobarbital for the patient. Under no conditions would the therapist be considered the "insurer" of good results, so that if he provided good care and the patient committed suicide anyway, the therapist would most probably not be held responsible should a suit develop.

The hospital, however, is in a more vulnerable position in that the failure to be adequately watchful of a suicidal patient is relatively easy to establish. If a patient is seriously suicidal the hospital can be expected to take special precautions such as locking the windows, doors and stairways, and under certain conditions applying physical and chemical restraints. Of course the recent emphasis on an "open door" policy in hospitals as a way to assist the patient to adjust to the outside world has to some extent decreased hospital liability for suicide. By the same token the hospital can be held liable despite an "open door" policy if it does not comply with its own requirements that there be sufficient personnel supervising the corridors. An example of this lack of precaution was seen in the *Havens* case, decided in 1962 by the Supreme Court of Washington (Benjamin vs Havens, Inc., 1962). In this case the hospital operated on the "open door" system, but for the protection of patients had a policy that a nurse would be stationed in the main corridor of the ward leading to an unlocked door or would be at least within close observation of that door.

The patient in this case was suffering from agitated depression and the therapist instructed that she be carefully watched. She had received several ECTs during the first ten days of hospitalization and had periods of depression and of sociability. One evening the patient ran down the main corridor through the unlocked outside door. She apparently injured herself when she fell through a hedge and down an embankment. The hospital was sued because there was no nurse guarding the corridor when this occurred, and it was a stated policy of the hospital that the main corridor would at least be within close observation of a nurse. In deciding this case the court held that the psychiatrist was not liable for the patient's injuries but that a jury could reasonably find negligence on the part of the hospital for not providing appropriate precautions.

The hospital is susceptible to a malpractice suit when it fails to exercise proper precautions consistent with the due care of suicidal patients, but like the therapist, the hospital cannot be viewed as an insurer of good results; it too must comply with a standard of appropriate hospital practice. When a patient unexpectedly jumps out of the tenth floor of a mental hospital or throws himself in front of a bus during a ward outing, the hospital could hardly be held responsible unless it could have forseen the event or been in a position to exert control and thus prevent the injury. And it must be realized that even in the face of the most careful precautions of known suicidal patients, there is no guarantee that the patient will not injure or kill himself.

Interestingly, most of the malpractice suits against hospitals involve the issue of failure to exert adequate therapeutic restraint of the patient. For the most part there have been virtually few if any successful suits against hospitals for using excessive restraints. (The exception to this would be a situation where unconventional restraints were used (Bellandi vs Park Sanitarium Association, 1931), when a tourniquet was applied to the neck of a patient and tightened resulting in cerebral ischemia and death.) Courts are inclined to favor any restraint thought necessary to protect patients and the public from uncontrollable behavior.

2) How could a no-fault system of medical malpractice be structured so as to include injuries that result from the negligence of health care institutions? There has been much discussion in the past few years about the failings of the current "fault" system for medical malpractice. The system is very expensive because of the occasional high settlements and because of the need for lawyers and considerable administrative activity. In addition a result of the fear of malpractice suits has been an incentive created for physicians, in particular, to practice defensive medicine by ordering expensive diagnostic procedures as a means of protecting themselves against the risk of a malpractice suit. Over and above the expense there has been little evidence that a jury trial actually provides information to the therapist that would help him to avoid adverse outcomes in the future and to assist him in achieving a higher quality of care. Finally, there is an inequity in the compensation system under the court process. Many injuries from therapeutic intervention go uncompensated, and only a very few receive exceptionally high awards by the court.

Alternatives have been proposed, such as using a system of arbitration whereby an expert rather than a jury would decide on disputes between therapists or hospitals and patients. This would avoid the need for long, expensive jury trials as well as the requirement in some cases for legal consultation. At the same time the arbiter has the legal power to determine blameworthiness, the cause of injuries and the extent of damages. In a study conducted by the Secretary's Commission on Medical Malpractice in 1973, four major arbitration plans were found operating in this country. Only a few cases had actually reached arbitration; many are settled by the patient and therapist, thereby avoid legal process. The use of arbitration and perhaps even screening panels to reduce the number of cases that would reach the courts with little likelihood of success in a trial need to be studied from the standpoint of fairness for all parties involved and from the perspective of the costs as compared to the existing court and jury system.

More effective in the long run might be the development of no-fault system of compensation that would operate automatically, like the automobile insurance system in states like Massachusetts, to compensate those injured by medical or psychiatric intervention. (This has been described in Chapter 16.) Briefly, it would be an adversity insurance system whereby patients incurring injury because of a diagnostic or treatment procedure in psychiatry, or because of an important omission in care, would be compensated for loss of wages and the medical or psychiatric expenses resulting from the injury. Psychiatric therapists would be required to identify adverse outcomes of patient care that probably could be avoided by appropriate prevention or treatment. If these outcomes occurred the patient would receive compensation automatically.

One of the significant advantages of this system of compensation is that it includes a mechanism for creating an incentive both for the therapist and the hospital to provide quality care. This would be accomplished by including a provision whereby the insurance policy of the therapist or hospital would be "experience-rated", that is, a provider with a loss experience higher than normal because of many adverse outcomes from his treatment would have his insurance premium for future years raised. When a patient is hospitalized it would be important to have it established which adverse outcomes should be paid for out of the psychiatric therapist's insurance policy and which should be the responsibility of the hospital. This decision would be based primarily on an evaluation as to which party was in the best position to avoid the incident that resulted in injury. The risk-bearer should therefore be the party that could have altered the situation and prevented the injury. For example, in the Havens case, clearly the hospital was in the position to add more personnel to the ward or to lock the corridor doors at times when the staff was minimal and thereby avoid the incident that led to injuries for the patient. Under other conditions where inappropriate medications are given or the patient suffers from severe adverse reactions from medicines, the therapist should be held responsible if he probably could have prevented the unfortunate outcome.

The concept of the no-fault system is at the present time highly theoretical. It appears that such a system could be applied to psychiatry in the same way it is applied to orthopedic surgery where one can more easily determine what is good care and what is obviously harmful. There would be major advantages in a no-fault system, both for the patient and the therapist. Besides being economically more efficient, it might also provide a better mechanism for inducing better quality of patient care, as well as avoiding the stigma attached to the therapist who is subjected to a malpractice action.

When an institution is grossly negligent or wilfully harmful, then, as in the case of therapists, the only appropriate recourse is the existing court process. Also, if an untoward outcome occurs that has not been identified as compensable but the patient feels could have been avoided, there would be a means, perhaps through arbitration or a regular trial, for determining if the insurance policy of the provider should pay for the losses of the patient.

REFERENCES

Bellandi vs Park Sanitarium Association, (1931) 214 Cal 472, 6 P 2d 508

Benjamin vs Havens, Inc, (1962) 60 Wash 2d 196, 373 P 2d 109

"The Best of Law and Medicine" (1968). Chicago, American Medical Association

Darling vs Charleston Memorial Hospital, (1965) 33 Ill 2d 326, 211 NE 2d 253; cert denied 383 US 946 (1966).

Davidson HA (1965): Forensic Psychiatry. New York, Ronald Press

Dawidoff DJ (1973): The Malpractice of Psychiatrists. Illinois, Charles C Thomas

Fiorentino vs Wenger, (1966) 26 App Div 2d 693, 272 NYS 2d 557

French vs Fisher, (1962) 50 Tenn App 587, 362 SW 2d 926

Havighurst CC, Tancredi LR (1973): Medical adversity insurance—a no-fault approach to medical malpractice and quality assurance. Health and Soc 51:125

Kapuschinsky vs United States, (1966) 248 F Supp 732 DSC.

Morse HN (1967): Psychiatric responsibility and tort liability. J Forensic Sci 12:305

Morse HN (1967): The tort liability of psychiatrists. Baylor Law Rev 19:208

Pederson vs Dumouchel, (1967) 431 P 2d 973

Perr R (1965): Liability of hospital and psychiatrist in suicide. Am J Psychiatry 122:631

Schwartz A (1971): Civil liability for causing suicide: A synthesis of law and psychiatry. Vanderbilt Law Rev 24: 217

Secretary's Commission on Medical Malpractice (1973): Report of the Secretary's Commission on Medical Malpractice. Washington, DC Department of Health Education and Welfare, Government Printing Office

Somers A (1969): Hospital Regulation: The Dilemma of Public Policy. New Jersey, Industrial Relations Section of Princeton University

Southwick R (1968): Hospital's responsibility. Cleveland–Marshall Law Rev 17:156

Tancredi LR, Woods J (1972): The social control of medical practice: Licensure versus output monitoring. Milbank Memorial Fund Quarterly 50:99

Tonsic vs Wagner, (1974) 329 A 2d 497

CONFLICTS IN RESPONSIBILITY ROLES OF THE **MENTAL HEALTH PROFESSIONAL**

19 RESPONSIBILITY
TO THE PATIENT

A psychiatric clinician may at times find himself caught in an ethical dilemma between serving the interests of his patients or those of society. While confidentiality is, of course, always an important aspect of the therapist–patient relationship, there are times when a clinician is told something in therapy and if he does not violate the confidence serious harm might come to the patient or to others. A patient may be planning to kill his spouse, children or some other person. Or perhaps he confesses a *fait accompli* to his psychotherapist out of guilt. Fortunately, in most circumstances when a patient discusses a desire to take his own or another's life, it is clear that he is telling his therapist because he wants to be controlled and protected from himself. It is usually, therefore, possible for a skilled therapist to persuade a violent patient to submit voluntarily to hospitalization and to a mutual alerting of relatives or other significant persons of his fear of loss of control over his impulses and his need for psychiatric care. Suicidal and homicidal patients, however, can be a source of anxiety and ethical conflict for the clinician when they do not voluntarily consent to hospitalization and consent cannot be readily obtained from concerned relatives or friends.

In this and the next chapter a few general considerations are raised that are pivotal in developing an understanding that transcends the specifics of individual case problems to what a clinician's responsibilities to his patients and to society at large should be.

PRIVACY

One consideration of particular importance is that of privacy. In the past, concern about privacy rights was restricted to alerting a physician that what transpired between him and his patient should not be passed on in conversations with families and friends. It also included avoiding the use of information obtained in a therapeutic encounter for financial gain, as through investments.

Today, the burgeoning of data banks threatens an individual's right to privacy. Many feel an existentialist *angst* as the advent of an Orwellian Big Brother era seems here. In countries such as Sweden, there is already such a highly integrated system of data collection that it is has been necessary to develop a Data Inspection Board to serve as a watchdog over the use of the immense amount of personal information collected for welfare purposes. A Swedish tradition backed by law has made the information generally available to the public. Such data which may alone seem innocuous could, if collected and put into devious hands, easily result not only in embarrassment for an individual but also possibly in his exploitation. For instance, that a woman has been recently widowed means little in itself; but if in addition to this she has inherited a great sum of money, subscribes to a number of romance magazines and tends to drink to excess, she could be exploited by an opportunist if he became aware of all these facts.

While the situation is not yet so grave in the United States, there is a growing amount of personal information that, if made generally available, could be used to an individual's detriment. More specifically, the policy that the records of hospitals be periodically reviewed has created a situation that has resulted in patients' medical and psychiatric case records being available to nonmedical individuals employed to review hospital records for completeness, treatment policies, *et cetera*. For some time insurance companies and employers have sought data to justify the payment of fees for medical services or compensation. While it is understandable that employers or insurance companies might not wish to pay great sums of money for psychiatric treatment when an ailment is one which the great majority of people can reasonably live with without medical intervention or with less costly forms of treatment, the intrusion into an individual's privacy remains disturbing.

Disclosure of personal information is especially injurious when it involves those who have been afflicted with one of the major psychiatric disorders. When a recent candidate for the vice-presidency of the United States was found to have a history of depression, we saw how the old stigma attached to mental illness was still very much a force. Former psychiatric patients are often alarmed to learn that the fact that they have been hospitalized for a psychiatric illness is not a secret, and become even more so to learn that their illness was labeled psychotic depression or schizophrenia.

One proposal to safeguard the right of privacy of personal information is that contracts be established between employers and insurance carriers so that an employer in no way may become involved in the processing of individual claims. This would not, of course, avert the problems that are created when an employer is also the insurance carrier nor does it avoid the problems that will be created if the government becomes involved with a health insurance policy. It is clear that the time has come for all clinicians concerned with psychiatric treatment to take a strong stand to protect their patients from an overly free system of information exchange or a situation may result that will significantly deter those suffering from psychiatric illness from obtaining the help that they need.

PSYCHIATRIC TESTIMONY

A psychiatrist's first responsibility is always the care of his patients. Good psychiatric care and societal goals should never be in conflict. Social institutions are created by men to help individuals both as individuals and in aggregates to achieve happiness and self-actualization. While these goals may be ambiguous, the steps toward achieving them are fairly clear. In psychiatry, this may be psychotherapeutic measures, organic therapy (*e.g.*, drugs, ECT) or social engineering so that the individual may return to functioning in a manner that will allow him to actualize as much of his potential as is possible without injury to himself or others in society.

Strictly speaking, it is not a psychiatrist's task to determine whether what has transpired in a patient's life makes him guilty of a crime; this is a matter to be decided by a jury. Providing recommendations for and the execution of an effective treatment plan is the primary task of the psychiatrist. It is always difficult, if not impossible, to say for certain that at the moment a crime was committed an individual was or was not culpable. Individual behavior is too complicated to allow anyone to make a definitive yes or no statement in such situations. What factors influence a court's decisions in such cases are known but still the psychiatrist must always realize that he can only express his humble opinion as to personal responsibility.

The use of a mental health clinician, in most instances a psychiatrist, as a legal witness has come under considerable scrutiny. It may be that psychiatric testimony should be limited until a verdict has been reached and then be given coupled with treatment recommendations. At the present time psychiatry can offer specific treatment recommendations for only a small proportion of those convicted of a crime. A person who in a manic state embezzles a fortune would fall in this genre. In general, however, psychiatry has little to offer in the treatment of criminals. There is still much to learn of the origins and control of aggressive and other criminal behavior.

With regard to civil suits, it may sometimes be necessary for a mental health professional to intercede to prevent the eliciting of information from a patient or his family which, while being immediately useful, may have long-term detrimental effects. One situation graphically demonstrates this point; a young woman, as a child, was coerced to testify in a divorce proceeding that her father had had intercourse with her. As a result he was imprisoned. Throughout her adolescence and young adult years, she was plaged by guilt, depression and suicidal ideation brought on by her father's accusations that it was her testimony that sent him to jail for several years. In such cases, a child should be protected and parents encouraged to use other means for obtaining a divorce.

BEHAVIORAL CONTROL

The converging factors which contribute to the development of psychiatric nosology (disease classification) are not always so objective and truly altruistic as the profession would like to pretend. Political and economic factors as well as one's own intrapsychic defensive structure contribute to how one determines what is normal or abnormal behavior. A review of the changing societal attitudes toward the use of various intoxicants such as alcohol and marijuana, as well as how medical, legal and ecclesiastical authorities have viewed various forms of sexual behavior from sex-role assignments to masturbation, divorce, birth control and homosexuality show how relative the concept is of what is psychopathological in our own and others' behavior. As discussed earlier in the text, there appear to be real psychiatric illnesses just like there are real medical illnesses, but these are few in number. Those behavioral aberrations which seem to be real illnesses tend to follow a medical model in their genetic patterns, course and treatment. Manic–depressive disease and depressive illness would be examples of this as well as, of course, the organic psychoses, (*e.g.*, psychosis with hyperthyroidism, brain tumor, *et cetera*). But the great number of behavioral aberrations such as the so-called neuroses, characterological disturbances and sexual deviations are more vague in their definition and even vaguer in how various people think they should be treated. Values, life philosophies and personal psychological defenses in these situations become entwined with objective medical evaluation.

With the recent advances in applied psychology, especially those based on learning theory, (*e.g.*, desensitization, aversive therapy, operant conditioning); psychosurgery, (*e.g.*, frontal lobotomy); and psychopharmacotherapy, (*e.g.*, the phenothiazines), there is justified concern over the ethical and legal aspects of behavioral control. The growing effectiveness of conditioning techniques and of the newer psychiatric medications makes it apparent that there now are methods of behavioral control which could be used to deprive a patient of the ability and right to make his own choices. This has in fact led some to believe that the psychiatric profession is involved in an attempt to prevent individual deviation from societal norms. Of course, the older therapies involving verbal techniques also appear to bring about some degree of behavioral change, but this is usually accomplished more slowly. In these circumstances the relatively gradual change allows a patient time to contemplate his moves and resist that which he may feel he doesn't want to change. The freedom in the long-term verbal psychotherapies may in fact be no greater than in the briefer chemotherapeutic or behavior therapies but the time differential may create that illusion. There is always a selective reinforcement of desired responses in any therapy. Ultimately a patient *in some way* comes to act as his therapist consciously or unconsciously feels he should.

Seymour Halleck (1974) has identified three areas in which the mental health profession should exert some control over the use of techniques for altering behavior. These are:

1. Those instances when a patient does not give his own verbal consent to being treated. While these generally involve civil or criminal commitment procedures, there may be situations in which treatments are imposed on voluntary patients without their cognizance.

2. Instances when a patient consents to treatment under duress. These include circumstances of commitment when punitive measures are threatened if a patient does not acquiesce to treatment, and cases of voluntary admission when family or community members threaten loss of love or status if a patient does not consent.

3. Those situations in which a patient consents to and may even ask for treatment. While one can conceive of ethical questions arising for the psychiatric practitioner even when patients request treatment, these are now the least controversial.

Halleck emphasizes the need for a truly "informed" consent when a patient is aware that he is psychotically ill. He also recognizes the need for safeguards in those situations when a patient cannot give consent but is obviously dangerous to himself or to others, when there is a reasonable probability that a treatment will benefit the patient as well as those around him and when the patient is incompetent to evaluate the necessity for treatment.

It is never ethically permissible to impose a treatment on a patient without at least giving him the opportunity to refuse it, provided that the patient is competent to do so. This condition would obviously make some forms of psychiatric research difficult; for instance, it would mean that it would be necessary to explain to a patient in a double-blind study that he may or may not be receiving an active drug as well as to warn him of the side effects as well as primary effects of all medications involved.

When a patient can understand what he is being treated for, there should be a full explanation of all treatments that are available and their advantages and disadvantages. If any side effects might result from treatment, these and their probability should be clearly explained. Under no circumstances should a special punishment be given if a patient refuses to be treated.

Finally, Halleck feels that under conditions when nonconsenting patients are given a treatment, the patient's treatment should be periodically reviewed and approved by a committee including at least one lawyer and a physician not directly involved in the patient's care.

The potential for abuse of behavioral modification without appropriate ethical or legal controls either from within the medical profession or from without (if that be the profession's choice) is that the individual can be rendered vulnerable by the "indiscriminate" use of conditioning as illustrated by the case of fifteen-year-old Alex in Anthony Burgess' nightmarish novel, *A Clockwork Orange.*

EFFECTIVENESS OF TREATMENT AND APPROPRIATENESS OF DIAGNOSIS

A major responsibility all mental health professionals have to their patients is to evaluate the effectiveness of various psychiatric treatment modalities. For some time it has been generally accepted that verbal psychotherapies were effective for a great number of psychiatric disorders. After all, it was argued, didn't people get better after spending several years in psychoanalysis? The question from a strictly scientific perspective is *not* whether an individual gets better after a given course of a treatment but rather would he improve more in one treatment than in another less costly one or improve more than if he had no treatment at all? This has been one of the more embarrassing questions in psychiatry. Often it is pushed aside by practicing clinicians who insist that psychological changes are subtle and that the instruments are too crude to pick up the fine changes that occur.

Hans Eysenck, a professor of psychology at the Maudsley Hospital in London, reported on a survey of evaluative studies of psychotherapy in the early 1950s. His report naturally drew comment and criticism from some circles, but overall it has been much respected; its conclusion that, in general, psychotherapy could not be demonstrated to be more efficacious than other treatment approaches and in some cases appeared no better than no treatment at all, gave rise to careful reconsideration of our traditional treatment approaches. The evaluation of any therapy, medical or psychological, is fraught with innumerable methodological problems such as appropriate selection of matched controls and control over other such variables as a change in social context which may influence behavior change. There are also variations in the clinician's individual skills and adeptness which are always lost in large studies. Some therapists are better treating one type of patient than another.

In addition, it appears that the theoretical framework for verbal therapy is not the important factor determining the success of treatment. Rather than a particular theoretical orientation, Freudian or Jungian psychoanalysis, for example, a factor or number of factors are common to the many types of therapy capable of producing a psychotherapeutic cure. One important factor in a cure or at least in the disappearance of symptoms seen in the course of many psychotherapies is the nature of the interpersonal bonds that make up a patient's social matrix as they operate both within a course of individual or group therapy as well as in his extratherapeutic relationships. When a person feels valued, loved and respected, be it among relatives and friends or in a therapy situation, he seems to do well, to be relatively happy, productive and less depressed.

The effects of the commonly used treatments of the major psychiatric illnesses are less equivocal. Studies of the use of electroshock and the tricyclic antidepressants and monoamine oxidase inhibitors in the treatment of depression, the use of lithium prophylaxis in manic–depressive disease and the phenothiazines in schizophrenia have demonstrated unequivocally the effectiveness of these treatment modalities in the acute, and in some cases chronic, treatment of these illnesses.

As clinicians, the questions one is ethically held responsible to ask about the treatments used for patients are:

1. Does the treatment work better than a less costly one, or better than no treatment at all?
2. Does the additional cost justify the use of one treatment that may be proved to be superior to another?
3. What is the long-term success of a treatment?

Although a patient may be better at the end of a given treatment, the course of the illness if left untreated may have been shorter than the treatment course. Therefore, one must know the natural history of a given psychiatric illness left untreated, and if a treatment appears successful even with this fact in mind does it help to prevent further episodes five, ten or fifteen years later?

Finally, it is incumbent upon psychiatric clinicians to see that their diagnoses are correct. The mislabeling of patients may lead to inappropriate treatments such as confinement, as well as contribute to a negative self-image. If a person is seriously, psychiatrically ill, his illness would be diagnosed and the appropriate treatment begun. If, however, he is a criminal and culpable for an illegal act, psychiatric labels should be secondary in the terms of disposition of the patient. Comparably, psychiatric diagnoses should not be used to maintain societal norms; they should suggest appropriate treatment. Terms such as "hysterical" or "homosexual" should be reserved to describe behaviors (in this case variations in sexual attitudes and expressions which relate to greater societal values) and not be considered psychiatric diagnoses or *prima facie* evidence of disease. Psychiatry has on occasion either willingly or not assumed the role previously assigned to religion as the guardian of societal norms of sexual morality in addition to its primary task of treatment of mental illness. Attitudes toward sex are culturally bound and what is "normal" at one period or in one sociocultural context may not be accepted in another.

Even if a patient has a real psychiatric illness such as manic–depressive disease, this diagnosis does not imply that he is dysfunctional in all areas. Although during periods of extreme mood swings it may be necessary to confine him to protect him or others, probably during most of his life he will be able to function quite normally in most situations.

LEGAL ASSISTANCE

Traditionally, psychiatry has limited its interventions to those disorders which may be described as psychological or psychosocial. Often patients turn to psychiatrists for problems that an accountant or lawyer should handle. A mental health professional should therefore have a heightened sensitivity to the legal and Constitutional rights of his patients. Not everyone is fortunate enough to know when he is being abused economically or otherwise and just what his legal rights are. This is particularly true of poor black and Puerto Rican groups who are frequently caught in a system they do not understand and do not know how to manipulate to their own advantage. It may be appropriate to have a lawyer for consultation or to act as a full-time staff member of a hospital to advise patients directly or by consultating their therapist. What may appear to be a depression with psychogenetic roots deep in a patient's past may hinge on the reality of his being unjustly and illegally abused of his rights or economically exploited. In such cases the appropriate treatment for his depression may not be antidepressant medication or psychotherapy but rather referral to a lawyer so that the issues involved may be clearly defined and his rights defended.

In addition to being available as counsel to patients, a staff lawyer would be an important adjunct to any psychiatric treatment facility to serve as consultant to mental health clinicians to inform them of the legal rights of patients, especially those being treated involuntarily. Problems that arise in such cases could immediately be handled in the best interests of both patient and therapist.

REFERENCES

Burgess A (1972): A Clockwork Orange. Middlesex, Penguin

Durkheim E (1951): Suicide: A Study in Sociology. New York, Free Press

Ennis B (1972): Prisoners of Psychiatry: Mental Patients, Psychiatry and the Law. New York, Harcourt, Brace and Jovanovich

Eysenck HJ, Rachman S (1965): The Causes and Cures of Neurosis. San Diego, RR Knapp

Halleck SL (1974): Legal and ethical aspects of behavioral control. Am J Psychiatry 131: 381–385

Klein DF, Davis JM (1969): Diagnosis and Drug Treatment of Psychiatric Disorders. Baltimore, Williams and Wilkins

Menninger K (1969): The Crime of Punishment. New York, Viking Press

Offenkrantz W, Tobin A (1974): Psychoanalytic psychotherapy. Arch Gen Psychiat 30: 593–606

Seglin MN (1974): Guarding the patient's right to privacy. Am Med News, March 11, 1974, p. 6

Slaby AE, Tancredi LR (In Press): Collusion for Conformity. New York, Jason Aronson

Wicker T (May 19, 1974): Checking Big Brother: II. The New York Times, p. 19

20 RESPONSIBILITY

TO SOCIETY

In the previous chapter the psychiatric clinician's responsibility to the patient was examined. The emphasis of the discussion was the belief that high quality treatment following appropriate diagnosis is not only valued as good medicine but also as an ethical goal. Such issues as safeguarding a patient's right to privacy and periodic evaluation of the efficiency and effectiveness of the various psychiatric treatment modalities must be an integral feature of a responsible treatment program in a medical situation, along with kindness and respect for the patient as a fellow human being. The behavioral control functions of psychiatry in particular have the danger of dehumanizing the patient and should be used only when there is strong treatment justification.

The use of psychiatry as a societal control agent cannot be dismissed easily. In this chapter another aspect of psychiatry, its responsibility to society, is scrutinized; major conflicts may arise for the professional who sees his primary function to be that of patient care. Should all of the mechanisms for controlling behavior in a society be invested in state police agencies? Or should some of the burden be shouldered by psychiatry? The obvious answer to this question is that in some circumstances psychiatry—because of its specialized knowledge of the genesis of aberrations of behavior—may be the preferred control instrument. This is particularly the case when a criminal act is performed by someone who has major psychopathology, such as paranoid schizophrenia, or a structural lesion of the brain that may result in violent and assaultive behavior. Clearly it is more appropriate for psychiatry to assume the control function, as members of this profession are more equipped to diagnose and treat these disturbances than are the police.

The issue becomes less clear though in other areas where individuals come into conflict with the law. While much has been written about sociopathic, psychopathic and criminal behavior in the annals of psychiatry, few objectively effective treatment recommendations have been proposed that have been used successfully to alter what most recognize to be common criminal behavior. Neurosurgical intervention does seem to be effective in treating some patients with lesions of the temporal lobe associated with violent behavior. Psychiatry has little definitive treatment for the great bulk of behavior that comes within the domain of legal authorities, such as robbery, theft, murder and rape. Various theories have been proposed for the psychogenesis of these behaviors, but these insights even if they are valid have certainly not contributed to any major reduction of crime.

The notion that psychiatry does have the tools for treating certain types of criminal behavior has gained considerable acceptance in recent years. As Kittrie (1971) points out in *The Right to Be Different,* there has been a decided shift away from the use of the criminal process to that of the therapeutic model in dealing with prevalent forms of victimless behavior, such as alcohol consumption and drug abuse, in addition to the injurious conduct of the sexual psychopath.

Kittrie's concern, however, has been that the therapeutic system is harsher on the individual, particularly when he has not engaged in conduct injurious to others, than if he were channelled through the criminal process. (In chapter five the legal pitfalls of such a system were pointed out.) Essential civil rights are conspicuously ignored when the individual is forced into a mental facility. The criminal process however is so structured as to place significant impediments in the way of law enforcement officers to minimize abuse of individual citizens. The adversary process has been shown to be an effective device for protecting the interests of all those involved in the determination of a socially unacceptable act. First the system provides a forum for the disclosure not only of the need for society to control certain behaviors but also of the circumstances surrounding the defendant which may have thrust him unwillingly into a "criminal" stance. Furthermore, by protecting the individual defendant against arbitrary decision-making on the part of those who represent the interests of society, the adversary system also serves the needs of society for stability and order.

In its present form the medical or psychiatric model does not offer significant protection against indiscriminate decision-making by societal control agencies. This is not to say that the trend toward interpreting many forms of victimless crime as evidence of an underlying psychiatric illness is necessarily incorrect but rather that by classifying such conduct as "illness," the chronic alcoholic and drug addict is thrust into a system almost totally insensitive to his rights as a citizen. The danger also exists that other varieties of human behavior not compatible with societal norms will also be viewed as evidence of "illness" with little medical justification. This would be an overt distortion of the major purpose of medicine which is treatment.

Perhaps, as suggested in the last chapter, it would be better if psychiatry limited itself to a description and exploration of the factors that contribute to what is described as criminal, sociopathic or psychopathic behavior. By limiting the present focus to these two tasks, there would be fewer confrontations between the psychiatric clinician and angry community members who feel that psychiatry has the knowledge base for therapeutic intervention in a group of situations and then become disillusioned when their expectations are not met. It seems premature to give psychopathic and sociopathic behavior the status of a "disease" based on the medical model. It is far likelier that the genesis of much crime lies in other factors such as the quality of the social matrix of a community, economic and educational opportunities and the presence of individuals in a child's development who serve as role models with values that are or are not consistent with those of the predominant subculture.

Now to turn to another responsibility of a psychiatric clinician—his patient's "right" to terminate his own life. A fairly cogent argument can be made that each person should have the freedom to take his own life; especially in cases of incurable illnesses such as terminal cancer, it would not only seem philosophically justifiable for an individual to end his own life, but it also might be in such an instance a profoundly kind act to let him do so. But what about a parent who is psychiatrically ill but not physically incurable. Does he have the right to make a decision to end his life considering the immediate and long-range consequences to the children? An immediate concern is how the children of the suicided parent will handle the immediate trauma, who will take care of the children's expenses or who will supply the warmth and nurturance that the children could have received from the parent had he recovered from his deep depression? Finally, there are the long-range effects on a child who feels he has been abandoned; some individuals never cease to ask themselves: "Why? Was it my fault? Was I a bad child? Didn't Mommy love me enough or didn't I love her enough?"

Experienced psychiatric professionals know that a family history of suicide increases the risk that a given patient will commit such an act. In addition, it is well documented that childhood loss through death, divorce or separation is a frequent antecedent of adult psychiatric problems. Therefore, even if it required forcible confinement, it would be a responsibility of the psychiatric clinician in such a situation to prevent the patient from taking his own life. This would be a responsibility to society, and particularly to a small segment of society—the patient's family.

Synoptically, one may reasonably state that the common interface of psychiatry and law *vis-a-vis* the greater society is the prevention of injury to other individuals and to the patient; psychiatry has an affirmative responsibility to protect both parties. On the other hand, neither medicine nor psychiatry as a specialty of medicine has an obligation to reinforce the moral value system of any one historical period by labeling acts as sick which produce minimal if any harm to an individual or to those with whom the individual interacts, anymore than the legal system should be used to give substance to a particular moral value system by labeling such acts "victimless crimes." Both medicine as a societal institution and psychiatry have been misused to reinforce contemporary standards of morality during various historical periods. A review of medicine's attitude toward abortion, masturbation and homosexuality is but an example of how society has used medicine to promulgate its views. Even divorce was at one time considered an indicant of psychopathology! At a time when an abortion was associated with serious complications and a high mortality rate, one can see how it would be incumbent upon a physician to protect his patients from these serious complications just as he would protect a patient from any other procedure that could result in serious harm or death. But today when the technique is relatively simple and performed under aseptic surgical conditions, it should clearly be the right of an individual woman to decide; she should not be made to feel immoral or to feel that she is denying her feminine role or maternal destiny, or to feel that she is a criminal. Comparably, a review of the descriptions of what contributes to or results from masturbation or homoerotic behavior found in older medical literature illustrates how the medical model was distorted to maintain varying societal concepts of morality.

Psychiatry should protect the individual's right to pursue what brings him personal happiness and self-actualization. Psychiatry should also protect society from *harmful* behavior, but not necessarily from all *deviant* behavior. Deviance is usually different from harmful conduct; for example, genius is clearly abnormal in a sense and therefore deviant from the norm. Creativity and innovation in artistic and intellectual pursuits as well as in individual human relationships require that a certain threshhold level of deviance be tolerated. Ironically, the protection of the individual's right for free expression which may go contrary to the predominant cultural ethic is another responsibility that psychiatry has to society. By protecting the individual's right to vary from traditional role assignment, the psychiatric clinician may serve to provide a milieu for the creative growth of many individuals who will eventually go on to make major contributions to society. This can be vividly illustrated by psychiatry's unique position in helping women, blacks and Puerto Ricans strive for goals which their parents considered unfathomable and totally inaccessible and against which great segments of the predominant subcultures set up barriers. For a long time the contributions that these segments of society could have made were forcibly kept at a minimum. The exact loss in terms of talent and innovation is inestimable.

The characterization of any behavior as "normal" or "appropriate" must always be qualified because it is from the extremes that would be deemed abnormal and behaviors which at one time may have been described as "inappropriate" that tomorrow's leaders and society's norms are found in their nascent form. To avoid the emergence of a one-dimensional, though well-adjusted and stable society, strong checks must be created to prevent an intolerant attitude toward nonconforming or aberrant behavior.

In keeping with the desired goal of maintaining a richly diversified society by restricting to some extent the forces for conformity, psychiatry must become aware of its potentiality for abuse, not only by psychiatric clinicians but by other segments in society. By describing some behaviors as healthy and others as sick, psychiatry creates a powerful linguistic tool which can be misused. Szasz (1970), in *Ideology and Insanity*, elucidates the extent to which psychiatric linguistics, terms like paranoid, projection and schizoid, can be used by various factions of society to objectively externalize others from the common stream of human experience, and thereby gain certain socioeconomic benefits. For example, at one time "nigger," "boy" and similar dehumanizing terms were used frequently as a way to demean and thereby to control the black population of this country. With the emergence of the civil rights movement in the early 1960s and a similarly strong surge of black power, these terms became rapidly unacceptable to the majority of the population and many began to reach for a different control apparatus, finding some relief for this purpose in psychiatric language. As a result it became common in the late 1960s and early '70s for terms like paranoid and sociopathic to be used to label blacks as well as other nonwhite minority groups in the population.

Psychiatry, therefore, is confronted with many ethical conflicts. Because of its basic inexactitude and its reliance on a constellation of behavioral manifestations as evidence of sickness, it presents a ready instrument for dehumanizing and abusing various minority groups in society. Most important, there is a shroud of mystery surrounding the field of psychiatry, an aura of omniscience which imputes greater authority to the language tool of the discipline than is warranted. As a result, terms like paranoid which are only vaguely understood by nonprofessionals are weighted with much more meaning than is justified by psychiatric knowledge.

Furthermore, such usage is distorted and applied indiscriminately for socioeconomic rather than medical reasons. Psychiatric terms are not only limited to racial or other societal control "needs," but in the business and political worlds psychiatry is having an increasingly important impact. Employers are often inclined to apply psychiatric characterizations to dissident or nonconforming employees and thereby justify impeding their career development.

In the field of politics the use of psychiatric terminology can be particularly devastating; the Eagleton incident during the 1972 presidential campaign boldly illustrates the destructive influence that psychiatric terminology can have on the success of a political candidate. On one level it might be argued strongly that psychiatry has an affirmative obligation to enter into the political arena by evaluating potential leaders. Perhaps the disclosure of appropriate psychiatric knowledge might have prevented the rise of Hitler. But the imprecision and vagueness of much psychiatric language allows it to be abused by psychiatrists and others in the political and social system.

There is little doubt that psychiatry is emerging as a powerful force for structuring society. At the present time, however, it is clouded by much mystery and subjective opinion which encourages a wide range of inaccuracies. The ethical responsibilities, therefore, for psychiatry are to educate the public not only about its strength as a therapeutic model, but also about the pitfalls which can render it a destructive force. The mystery of psychiatry which seems to facilitate its curative role at the same time imbues it with an authority which is not only inappropriate but dangerous to society. The myth element of psychiatry must be shown to be just that—myth—before the precision of terms essential for high quality diagnosis and treatment can be achieved. This process will not only be immensely beneficial to the discipline itself but will inevitably benefit many by removing a powerful and easily distorted tool for controlling society.

REFERENCES

Kittrie N (1973): The Right To Be Different. Baltimore, Johns Hopkins Press
Slaby AE, Tancredi LR (In Press): Collusion for Conformity. New York, Jason Aronson
Szasz T (1970): Ideology and Insanity. New York, Doubleday
Szasz T (1972): Law, Liberty and Psychiatry. New York, Collier Books
Szasz T (1973): Mental illness as a metaphor. Nature 242:305

21 REALIGNMENT
OF ROLES

The primary function of psychiatry is that of the care of patients. There can be no argument with this statement, for psychiatry, like other medical specialties, has evolved out of a tradition whose origins are in the Hippocratic Oath which emphasizes that the interests and needs of the patient be paramount in the physician's mind. The corollary of this would be the command that the physician must not in any way induce harm to the patient.

Since the breakdown of ecclesiastical law in Europe which was directed primarily at determining the appropriateness of various forms of human behavior, unlike the other specialties in medicine psychiatry has assumed two functions. It is first concerned with the mental health of disturbed patients; but it is also involved with societal control functions which can work counter to the interests of patients. In this latter respect, psychiatry and law are similar as they are both invested in perhaps different ways with the responsibility of defining the limits of what society will accept in relationships among persons and institutions. Law is primarily involved with acts that inflict definite evils or harm. It is concerned, therefore, with the outcomes of acts which are injurious to others or to self, if injuring one's self damage to society results.

Psychiatry focuses on the manifestations of behavior rather than the outcomes of that behavior. Using the medical model based on the distinction between sickness and health, psychiatry characterizes certain forms of behavior as evidence of illness—for example, suicide, prostitution, sexual deviance and drug usage. The reasons for such classifications may be open to question. On one hand, the argument is strong that some behavior is clearly suggestive of mental illness. The catatonic patient who sits in the corner of a room for hours and days without controlling even elementary biological functions is understandably considered mentally ill. But as we examine behaviors which are classified as sicknesses according to psychiatric nosology, the strength of the argument for such descriptions may not be purely medical. Psychiatry unlike other forms of medicine has few real principles on which it can rely for objectively distinguishing between sickness and health. It becomes influenced, therefore, by societal notions and preferences regarding human behavior. Where psychiatry adheres strictly to a definition of illness that points directly at psychological or physiological dysfunction, it is complying with the purest tradition of medicine in classifying disease. If the classification veers away from one based on dysfunction, then psychiatric nosology becomes influenced by societal perceptions of "normal" or appropriate behavior. When the latter occurs, psychiatry is entering into a control function in addition to its medical role.

The effects of psychiatry in the control of human behavior are complicated. Psychiatry both influences what the criminal law treats as criminal—for example, many forms of sexual "deviance" such as homosexuality—and subjects to medical controls activities that are not classified as criminal; for example, promiscuous heterosexual behavior in women, minor acts of masochism and fetishism and even withdrawal or isolation though not controlled under any existing laws are strongly discouraged by psychiatry which views such behavior as evidence of illness or dysfunction, thereby reflecting social values to a great extent. The combined effects of law and psychiatry, therefore, achieve a profound impact on controlling a wide range of socially undesirable behavior. By assuming a role in social control, psychiatry aids the law in carving away at individual privacy and freedom of expression even in cases where there is no objective evidence of harm to others.

Psychiatry's role in social control has been increasing over the past years despite the warnings by many scholars such as Szasz and Kittrie who warn of the dangers to individual freedom of using a sickness model for social control. The shift from the legal model, that is, designating certain conduct as criminal, to the psychiatric model for control is closely tied to the question of personal responsibility for one's behavior. To label an offender criminal there must usually be evidence to show he was responsible for his actions. In the past virtually everyone including the insane was held responsible for his actions. With the advent of formalized tests for insanity starting primarily with the M'Naghten Rule, a gradual narrowing of the concept of personal responsibility has taken place. As seen in chapter one, the definition of insanity for a defense against murder has broadened considerably over the past hundred years. So likewise has there been increasing application of the notion that the individual under many circumstances is not in full control of his actions.

Many new classes of individuals from alcoholics and drug addicts to the sexual psychopath are thought to lack the capacity to be responsible for their behavior. As a result, the legal system with its court trials and punitive measures, such as fines and imprisonment, is no longer viewed as the appropriate disposition for a vast array of offenders. More reliance is placed on psychiatry to "treat" instead of "punish," and thereby to control more effectively those who deviate from society's standards. With this trend away from attributing personal responsibility for conduct, psychiatry becomes empowered with significant societal control functions which create in many cases a conflict of interest in the psychiatrist who is primarily concerned with the medical needs of his patient but is also the societal agent mandated to control unacceptable and deviant conduct.

Psychiatry controls behavior in two ways. It can be a direct control, as through commitment of patients for treatment, or it can be an indirect control, that is, by reflecting societal values in the way it classifies mental illnesses.

Direct Societal Control

We have already seen that the psychiatrist has the significant power to confine those whom he feels require psychiatric treatment. The laws in the states vary concerning the extent of power the psychiatrist has. In some states the reasons for commitment are narrowly defined, often requiring that the patient be either harmful to himself or to others. Other states, however, have an expanded provision for commitment, allowing the psychiatrist to commit those whom he feels would benefit from mental health therapy. Such a provision is essentially all-inclusive with minimal qualifications, leaving the decision as to whether confinement is warranted up to the psychiatrist. Whereas many states allow commitment primarily for the severely mentally ill, there is a trend toward permitting involuntary commitment of other persons who might have otherwise been handled through the legal system. The chronic alcoholic, drug addict and certain psychosexual offenders are susceptible to commitment in much the same way as are psychotic patients should the psychiatrist decide that therapy is required. In some states the preferred route for disposition of those who break the laws against alcoholism and drug abuse is the medical care system, and in particular, psychiatric therapy.

Along with direct control through commitment is the growing involvement of psychiatry in the determination of responsibility for conduct. The court frequently calls upon the psychiatrist to assess whether an offender of societal rules should be held responsible for his conduct. The issue at stake is whether or not such individuals possess the capacity to understand what they have done, both intellectually and emotionally, and to have controlled their behavior. The psychiatrist is placed in the pivotal position of assisting in the decision of culpability for criminal acts.

One additional form of direct control is that of the use of psychiatry for political purposes. This is not presently of any significance in this country, but there have been many episodes of the use of psychiatry for control of political dissidence in other countries, Russia in particular. The recent Mendevev affair is one such example. A renowned geneticist, Zhores Mendevev, was suddenly removed from his home and confined to a psychiatric institution. The authorities in Russia alleged that he was insane; however, there was no evidence of this from his behavior prior to commitment. It was learned upon his release that he was confined because of his controversial views regarding government activities.

Indirect Societal Control

In its classification of mental illness psychiatry has been influenced by societal notions of personality deformity. Psychiatry has inculcated the values and norms of society by classifying such behaviors as sexual deviancy, marijuana usage and suicide as illnesses. There is little doubt that some individuals engaging in sexual deviancy might also suffer conflicts in their personality. At the same time, however, the behavior itself can hardly be considered equivalent to a disease condition. The issue of primary importance for determining mental illness is the extent to which conflicts arise around behavior that might impede the normal functioning of the individual and prevent his ultimate personal fulfillment. The fact that one is a homosexual does not *per se* describe the extent to which he can adjust to reality and achieve happiness.

In *Portrait of a Marriage* Nigel Nicolson describes the marriage arrangement of his famous parents, Vita Sackville-West and her husband, Harold Nicolson. This couple experienced a long-term, intense relationship in spite of the fact that both participated in heterosexual and homosexual experiences outside of marriage. If the author's portrayal is reliable, the couple had a significant and enduring relationship which, unlike many marriages, seemed to intensify in its later years.

Except in the case of psychotics, the manifestation of behavior, particularly when other individuals are not victims, should not be the important characteristic for determining the existence of a mental disorder. In designating behavior *per se* as mental illness, psychiatry serves the role of legitimizing the control of individuals whose activities are not in conformance with prevailing social norms. Such control can occur through the legal process which is influenced by psychiatry's classification of inappropriate social behavior as sickness. By providing a medical reason for controlling such behaviors as consenting homosexuality, suicide or marijuana usage, the law can rationalize its control of such actions by pointing to the need for preventing harm to the individual participating in the behavior. Where crimes do not involve victims, the law often points to the vague and unproven effect that certain conduct may have on the society's stability. The reason for cautioning against the use of psychiatry for classifying certain behaviors as illness is that it results in a distortion of the societal role of psychiatry. It should not be an instrument for controlling behavior which is deemed inappropriate, but rather psychiatry should classify diseases on the basis of objective criteria, such as the effects that such behavior has on the adjustment, stability and happiness of the individual. The sexual deviant may experience as authentic a relationship as a comparable partner in a heterosexual union.

With regard to homosexuality, it is interesting that the American Psychiatric Association has recently removed such behavior from its classification of mental diseases. Many feel that homosexuality should never have been classified as a mental disease; however, when the decision was made to classify homosexuality as a disease, it was considered to be repulsive behavior by the majority of the population. In recent years the attitude to homosexuality has changed considerably. With present-day requirements for zero population growth, there is no longer the incentive to control sexual behaviors that do not result in children. As a consequence of this and also due to strong vocal interest groups such as the Mattachine Society, there has been a trend toward greater acceptance of homosexuality and other forms of sexual deviancy. The point of particular interest in this discussion is that the American Psychiatric Association has essentially deleted homosexuality from its classification of mental illnesses at the time that homosexuality gained significant acceptance by the majority of the population. This fact alone demonstrates the influence that societal norms and values have on the classifications of mental illness.

In effect, then, the medical model has been used to affirm societal notions about appropriate conduct and thus to control behavior which does not meet with societal approval. In most cases this is an indirect control; that is, the designating of certain deviant behaviors as sickness discourages many from participating in these kinds of activities and influences the extent to which those engaging in deviancy are able to achieve fulfillment. There is an element of a self-fulfilling prophecy in the psychiatric classification of certain conduct as illness. Though it may be argued that the manifestation of behavior in itself should not be the principal basis for classifying mental disease, the labeling of such behavior as illness actually induces a sickness role or attitude in many who have chosen a deviant life-style. The control is direct in the psychiatric classification of victimless behavior as mental illness supports and often gives impetus to the legal decisions to classify such conduct as criminal. Hence, in most of the states in this country, sodomy, homosexuality and marijuana usage are listed in the criminal codes.

Psychiatry's role in societal control is not completely without merit. Certainly in the case of the severely ill psychotic who on an emergency admission clearly demonstrates the desire to inflict harm on others or on himself there is justification for investing psychiatrists with limited control capabilities. The concept of short-term psychiatric confinement for observation purposes with early involvement of the legal system to assure the rights of patients seems quite sound from the standpoint of the patient as well as that of society. It is perhaps in those instances when patients suffer from severe psychoses and are also potentially harmful that there is the most meaningful integration of psychiatric knowledge with the need for societal control. Even under these conditions, however, patients must be protected from the abuses of power common in mental hospitals. The safeguarding of the rights of patients might be achieved by providing legal representation in the mental health institution so that patients can have immediate access to legal advice and assistance. States such as New York have already developed a system for legal representation in their mental health hospitals. Beyond this some states require that patients who have been committed, especially involuntarily committed, be reviewed frequently so that their confinement status can be altered quickly should there be a major improvement in their mental condition.

Except in those emergency circumstances where the psychotic and dangerous patient must be immediately confined, the psychiatrist should divest himself of societal control functions. To accomplish this, it will be necessary to reconceptualize the notion of mental disease.

Perhaps the most appropriate role, therefore, of the psychiatrist and mental health worker would be that of an advisor to the legal system, thereby assuring that the power for control remains in the hands of legal authorities who are regulated closely by provisions which protect citizens from abuses against their Constitutional rights.

In addition to divesting itself of most of its societal control functions, psychiatry should also reassess the capacities of various groups of the mentally ill to execute certain legal functions. The issue of determining whether or not a patient can be held responsible for his actions is a difficult one. As seen in the discussion of the insanity defense the concept of responsibility for criminal action is ill defined. When considering one's civil rights, such as the right to enter into business contracts and marriages and the right to manage personal property, the notions of cognitive capacity and responsibility become even more perplexing. It might be safe to say that just because a patient is confined to a mental institution does not necessarily mean that he cannot perform some of these tasks. A paranoid schizophrenic may not be capable of understanding that he has not been singled out by others to be persecuted, but he may well be capable of handling his financial matters. But most of the states in this country deny those who have been committed, particularly if involuntarily committed, most of their decision-making prerogatives over personal property.

Psychiatry should once again be put into the position of justifying why certain classes of patients are denied specific legal rights. It may be that, on reflection, many who are not now allowed to conduct their personal affairs should be granted this power. The capacity to function in one area of life may not necessarily be related to the capacity to perform other tasks. Therefore, it is important that there be a closer association between illnesses and the faculty for executing certain legal functions. The use of the sickness–health model has created many assumptions regarding patients which are probably no longer justified on the basis of current psychiatric knowledge. Simply because a patient is labeled ill does not mean one should leap to the conclusion that he is too irresponsible to be expected to make a valid will or to manage his business affairs.

By divesting itself of societal control functions, and by becoming more finely tuned to the relationship between mental illness and responsibility, psychiatry will be more intimately aligned with the other disciplines in medicine. Involvement in the legal system will be limited to cases in which psychiatry is capable of providing objectively derived information regarding the capacity of specific patients to understand their conduct or to participate in their personal business transactions.

In addition to the need for redefining the role of psychiatry it is also important to consider the legal implications of the greater responsibility that is being given to paraprofessionals in psychiatry. As psychiatric nurses and social workers assume more significant roles in patient care, they will also be exposed to many of the legal issues which now confront only psychiatrists; for example, the issues of confidentiality of information and psychiatric malpractice are already applicable to some degree to mental health workers in general. The divestment of societal control functions is particularly crucial at this time as other professionals are beginning to assume the legal powers previously reserved for psychiatrists alone. Psychiatric social workers operating under the supervision of psychiatrists are often the key personnel who decide the appropriateness of involuntary commitment. Similarly, psychiatric nurses and social workers exert powerful influences on deciding when treatment and particularly hospitalization should be terminated.

REFERENCES

Chayet NL (1968): Legal neglect of the mentally ill. Am J Psychiatry 125:785–792

Editorial note (on Zhores Mendevev) (August 20, 1973): Time, p. 332

Kittrie N (1971): The Right to Be Different: Deviance and Enforced Therapy. Baltimore, Johns Hopkins Press

Mayer EJ (1969): Lawyer in a mental hospital. Ment Hyg 53:14–16

Nicolson N (1973): Portrait of a Marriage. New York, Atheneum

Slaby AE, Tancredi LR (In Press): Collusion for Conformity. New York, Jason Aronson

Szasz T (1963): Law, Liberty and Psychiatry. New York, Macmillan

ADDENDA

TO CHAPTERS 4 and 5

The United States Supreme Court has recently reviewed the Donaldson case*
and held on 26 June 1975 that patients cannot be confined in mental institutions
involuntarily and without treatment if they are able to survive in society and if they
are not dangerous to anyone.[†] This decision is geared to protecting those who are
institutionalized simply for custodial reasons because they are impoverished,
eccentric, old, or unwanted, though in fact harmless and able to function on the
outside. The Court stated that mental illness is insufficient in itself to justify
confining these patients. In effect the Court decided that if patients are capable of
surviving on the outside and are not dangerous and not receiving treatment, then
there is no justification for their confinement in an institution. It did not, however,
resolve two important related constitutional issues, i.e., 1) whether those who are
not dangerous and are able to function on the outside can be confined unwillingly
for the purpose of receiving treatment, and 2) whether those who are mentally ill
and dangerous have a right to be treated when confined involuntarily.

*Case #74-8. O'Connor v. Donaldson (decided June 26, 1975).
[†]"High Court Curbs Power to Confine the Mentally Ill." The New York Times, June 27, 1975.
P. 1, column 5 and p. 36, column 33.

TO CHAPTER 6

The Supreme Court of California recently made a decision that could seriously
undermine the trust relationship between therapist and patient (Tarasoff vs Regents
of University of California, 1974*). The court said in effect that if a therapist
believes, on the basis of his professional skill in treating a patient, that a warning
is necessary to prevent danger to another, he is "legally obligated" to give
appropriate warning.[†] Besides placing the therapist in the very difficult position of
deciding the validity of his patient's threats, in order to avoid being sued for
carelessly disclosing confidential information, this court decision could deter people
from seeking treatment, or at least from making full and free disclosure of their
thoughts.

*Tarasoff vs Regents University of California, (1974) 118 California Reporter 129
[†]"Potential victims must be told of danger from violent patients." Clinical Psychiatry News. 3:1
(February 1975)

Because of the implications of this decision regarding the viability of psychotherapy, the California Supreme Court has been asked to reconsider its decision and has agreed to do so. If it decides to let the decision stand, efforts will probably be made by various professional interest groups to bring about legislative action in California to counteract the decision. Otherwise the decision could be appealed to the U.S. Supreme Court to determine its constitutionality. As it now stands, the decision is operative only in California.

INDEX

75 76 77 78 79   9 8 7 6 5 4 3 2 1